Sports Related Foot & Ankle Injuries

Editor

PAUL R. LANGER

CLINICS IN PODIATRIC MEDICINE AND SURGERY

www.podiatric.theclinics.com

Consulting Editor
THOMAS ZGONIS

April 2015 • Volume 32 • Number 2

ELSEVIER

1600 John F. Kennedy Boulevard • Suite 1800 • Philadelphia, Pennsylvania, 19103-2899

http://www.theclinics.com

CLINICS IN PODIATRIC MEDICINE AND SURGERY Volume 32, Number 2
April 2015 ISSN 0891-8422, ISBN-13: 978-0-323-35984-9

Editor: Jennifer Flynn-Briggs
Developmental Editor: Casey Jackson

Clinics in Podiatric Medicine and Surgery (ISSN 0891-8422) is published quarterly by Elsevier Inc., 360 Park Avenue South, New York, NY 10010-1710. Months of issue are January, April, July, and October. Business and Editorial Offices: 1600 John F. Kennedy Blvd., Ste. 1800, Philadelphia, PA 19103-2899. Customer Service Office: 3251 Riverport Lane, Maryland Heights, MO 63043. Periodicals postage paid at NewYork, NY and additional mailing offices. Subscription prices are $305.00 per year for US individuals, $450.00 per year for US institutions, $155.00 per year for US students and residents, $370.00 per year for Canadian individuals, $544.00 for Canadian institutions, $435.00 for international individuals, $544.00 per year for international institutions and $220.00 per year for Canadian and foreign students/residents. To receive student/resident rate, orders must be accompanied by name of affiliated institution, date of term, and the *signature* of program/residency coordinator on institution letterhead. Orders will be billed at individual rate until proof of status is received. Foreign air speed delivery is included in all *Clinics* subscription prices. All prices are subject to change without notice. POSTMASTER: Send address changes to *Clinics in Podiatric Medicine and Surgery*, Elsevier Health Sciences Division, Subscription Customer Service, 3251 Riverport Lane, Maryland Heights, MO 63043. **Customer Service: 1-800-654-2452 (US). From outside of the US, call 314-447-8871. Fax: 314-447-8029. E-mail: JournalsCustomerService-usa@elsevier.com (for print support); JournalsOnlineSupport-usa@elsevier.com (for online support).**

Reprints. For copies of 100 or more of articles in this publication, please contact the Commercial Reprints Department, Elsevier Inc., 360 Park Avenue South, New York, NY 10010-1710. Tel.: 212-633-3874; Fax: 212-633-3820; E-mail: reprints@elsevier.com.

Clinics in Podiatric Medicine and Surgery is covered in *MEDLINE/PubMed (Index Medicus)* and *EMBASE/Excerpta Medica*.

Contributors

CONSULTING EDITOR

THOMAS ZGONIS, DPM, FACFAS
Professor and Director, Externship and Reconstructive Foot and Ankle Fellowship Programs, Division of Podiatric Medicine and Surgery, Department of Orthopaedics, University of Texas Health Science Center San Antonio, San Antonio, Texas

EDITOR

PAUL R. LANGER, DPM, ABPM, FAAPSM
President, American Academy of Podiatric Sports Medicine; Twin Cities Orthopedics, Edina; Adjunct Clinical Faculty, Department of Family Practice, University of Minnesota Medical School, Minneapolis, Minnesota

AUTHORS

MAGALI FOURNIER, DPM, FACFAS
Departments of Orthopaedics, Podiatry and Sports Medicine, Gundersen Health Systems, LaCrosse, Wisconsin

BRIAN W. FULLEM, DPM, FAAPSM, FACFAS
Private Practice: Elite Sports Podiatry, Clearwater, Florida

FAYE E. IZADI, DPM
Seal Beach Podiatry Group Inc, Seal Beach, California

DAVID W. JENKINS, DPM, FACFAS, FAAPSM
Midwestern University Fellow, President of the American Academy of Podiatric Sports Medicine, Regional Clinical Advisor for the Healthy Athletes FIT FEET Program United States Special Olympics, Podiatric Consultant for the Los Angeles Dodgers, Professor, Arizona School of Podiatric Medicine, College of Health Sciences, Midwestern University, Glendale, Arizona

ALEX KOR, DPM, MS
Department of Orthopaedic Surgery, The Johns Hopkins University, Baltimore, Maryland

R. CLINTON LAIRD, DPM, FAAPSM, FACFAS
Port Charlotte, Florida

PAUL R. LANGER, DPM, ABPM, FAAPSM
President, American Academy of Podiatric Sports Medicine; Twin Cities Orthopedics, Edina; Adjunct Clinical Faculty, Department of Family Practice, University of Minnesota Medical School, Minneapolis, Minnesota

DOUGLAS H. RICHIE, DPM, FACFAS, FAAPSM
Seal Beach Podiatry Group Inc, Seal Beach, California

Contents

This article reviews the history of sports medicine highlighting the "jogging boom" of the 1970s and the advocacy of Dr George Sheehan, which boosted the position of podiatry in sports medicine. Significant events in mainstream sports medicine that promoted the rise of podiatric medicine are discussed. Reasons as to why podiatric medicine should be a member of the sports medicine team are outlined, and lastly, examples that highlight podiatric medicine as participants alongside other specialties in the evaluation and care of athletes are given.

Some common overuse injuries, such as Achilles tendinopathy and plantar fasciitis (or fasciopathy), can be refractory to treatment. When standard treatment options fail, operative intervention often becomes the treatment of last resort. Recently, newer technologies have been developed and refined, and can provide potential benefits for these conditions using noninvasive and minimally invasive approaches. Two technologies, extracorporeal shock wave therapy and ultrasound-guided percutaneous tenotomy/fasciotomy are discussed.

The ankle sprain is the most common injury in sport and has a high incidence of long-term disability. This disability may be partly due to early return to sport before ligament healing has been completed. The podiatric physician can follow sound guidelines for making a return-to-play decision for athletes suffering from an ankle sprain. The decision-making process requires the podiatric physician to monitor the rehabilitation process and then administer patient self-reported questionnaires as well as functional performance tests to assess the status of ankle function after injury.

Clinical diagnostic tests objectively evaluate lower extremity ailments of the athlete. The positive squeeze test is found to be reproducible for ankle syndesmotic injury but is a poor prognosticator. The anterior drawer and talar tilt tests assess lateral ankle sprains. These have limitations secondary to positioning and guarding by the athlete, so comparison with the asymptomatic extremity is recommended. The Ottawa ankle rules assess possible fractures of the ankle and midfoot. The Thompson test evaluates Achilles tendon tears, whereas the windlass technique and the modified Lachman test examine the integrity of the plantar fascia and metatarsophalangeal joint capsule.

Forefoot and midfoot injuries in the athlete are common. Injuries of the digits include subungual hematomas and fractures. Metatarsal fractures occur frequently in sports, and their treatments range greatly. Hyperflexion and extension injuries about the first metatarsophalangeal joint can be very debilitating. Midfoot sprains and fractures require a high index of suspicion for diagnosis.

When athletes train harder the risk of injury increases, and there are several common overuse injuries to the lower extremity. Three of the most common lower extremity overuse injuries in sports are discussed including the diagnosis and treatments: medial tibal stress syndrome, iliotibial band syndrome, and stress fractures. The charge of sports medicine professionals is to identify and treat the cause of the injuries and not just treat the symptoms. Symptomatology is an excellent guide to healing and often the patient leads the physician to the proper diagnosis through an investigation of the athlete's training program, past injury history, dietary habits, choice of footwear, and training surface.

Life spans are increasing and research is showing more and more how important exercise is to successful aging. Medical practitioners need to appreciate the physiologic and physical changes that occur with age, as well as the significant benefits of physical activity, so they not only can properly treat their older patients but also so they can promote the benefits of exercise to their sedentary older patients.

Rehabilitation of an athlete can present its own challenges. Few protocols are available to guide physicians in proper return to sport. Rehabilitation after foot and ankle sport injury can be categorized into 3 different stages but should also be individualized. The focus of this article is to help the treating physician in creating a protocol to safely return an injured athlete back to sport based on current literature and principles.

CLINICS IN PODIATRIC MEDICINE AND SURGERY

Foreword

Sports Related Foot and Ankle Injuries

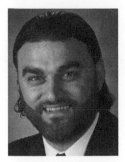

Thomas Zgonis, DPM, FACFAS
Consulting Editor

This issue of *Clinics in Podiatric Medicine and Surgery* is focused on the diagnosis and treatment of sports-related foot and ankle injuries. A variety of topics from acute osseous and soft tissue injuries to overuse lower extremity injuries and rehabilitation are very well covered by our guest editor, Dr Langer, and invited authors. Special attention is emphasized in treating the competitive athlete as well as the physically active older individuals and aging athletes.

In this issue, the guest editor, Dr Langer, and the invited authors have done an excellent job in addressing some of the most common podiatric sports medicine pathologies that can be used as a great reference to our readers. I thank you again for your outstanding submissions.

Thomas Zgonis, DPM, FACFAS
Externship and Reconstructive Foot & Ankle Fellowship Programs
Division of Podiatric Medicine and Surgery
Department of Orthopaedics
University of Texas Health Science Center San Antonio
7703 Floyd Curl Drive–MSC 7776
San Antonio, TX 78229, USA

E-mail address:
zgonis@uthscsa.edu

Clin Podiatr Med Surg 32 (2015) xi
http://dx.doi.org/10.1016/j.cpm.2015.01.002
0891-8422/15/$ – see front matter © 2015 Published by Elsevier Inc.

podiatric.theclinics.com

Preface

Sports Related Foot and Ankle Injuries

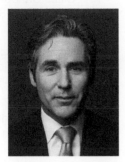

Paul R. Langer, DPM, ABPM, FAAPSM
Editor

This issue of *Clinics in Podiatric Medicine and Surgery* is focused on sports medicine, with a range of topics that have clinical significance but also provide relevant and timely information on topics important to our patients like aging and public health. Today sports medicine is much more than just treating competitive athletes. Due to increasing sports participation, increasing life spans, and growing knowledge about the benefits of an active lifestyle, sports medicine practitioners are treating patients with very diverse activity levels, age ranges, and athletic abilities. Along with this changing athletic population, the subspecialty of podiatric sports medicine continues to evolve as research accumulates, technology improves, and the demand for sports medicine services increase.

A sports medicine podiatrist does not function in isolation within their clinic and needs to keep abreast of the latest information. They need to interact with athletes in training rooms, at athletic events, and in conjunction with coaches and other members of the patient's medical team. Because of this, providers need to be well-versed in the latest philosophies and techniques regarding exam, treatment, and technology. Aging athletes and those seeking to improve their health through athletics will continue to become a bigger segment of the sports medicine patient population, and there are special considerations for these individuals. Sports medicine practitioners can and should not only treat injured athletes but also educate their patients on the importance of maintaining an active lifestyle.

The contributing authors are all experienced, respected sports medicine practitioners and, not coincidentally, active and athletic individuals themselves. Their collective knowledge and experience were sought out in order to provide the reader with the most comprehensive, up-to-date, and evidence-based information possible.

Clin Podiatr Med Surg 32 (2015) xiii–xiv
http://dx.doi.org/10.1016/j.cpm.2015.01.001
0891-8422/15/$ – see front matter © 2015 Published by Elsevier Inc.

podiatric.theclinics.com

Every athlete and active individual wants to heal and return to their activity as quickly as possible. Podiatrists have a unique and valuable perspective as sports medicine practitioners and can provide the expertise that can help athletes achieve their goals.

Paul R. Langer, DPM, ABPM, FAAPSM
Twin Cities Orthopedics
2010 West 65th Street
Edina, MN 55435, USA

Adjunct Clinical Faculty
Medical School
University of Minnesota
Minneapolis, MN, USA

E-mail address:
paullanger@tcomn.com

The Podiatrist as a Member of the Sports Medicine Team

David W. Jenkins, DPM, FACFAS, FAAPSM

KEYWORDS

- Sports medicine • American Academy of Podiatric Sports Medicine
- Team podiatrist • Multidisciplinary sports medicine clinic

KEY POINTS

- This article reviews the history of sports medicine from Biblical times up until the late 1960s.
- In the 1970s, the "jogging boom" and the advocacy of Dr George Sheehan put podiatric medicine on the map with regards to sports medicine.
- Significant interdisciplinary sports medicine conferences, publication of popular mainstream books on running injuries, and the formation of the American Academy of Podiatric Sports Medicine further promoted the rise of podiatric medicine.
- The appointment of podiatric physicians to positions such as Team Podiatrist for professional sports teams and members of the medical team for the Olympic Games confirms podiatric medicine as a major player in sports medicine.
- A description of what an interdisciplinary sports medicine team might look like is provided. The typical members are listed and the pros and cons of such a team are described.
- Rationale as to why podiatric medicine should be a member of the sports medicine team is given, as well as actual examples of such collaboration.

INTRODUCTION

Writing a dissertation on *The Podiatrist as a Member of the Sports Medicine Team* presented several barriers, primarily of which is the paucity of information on said topic. In no way was the search for information comparable with a topic such as *Advances in Achilles Tendon Rehabilitation*, where the medical literature and associated evidence is robust.

It is pertinent to warn the reader that much of what follows is anecdotal and based on the author's experiences and observations in the world of podiatric sports medicine. These experiences are substantial, in part, because the author began his career

Disclosure: None.
Arizona School of Podiatric Medicine, College of Health Sciences, Midwestern University, 19555 North 59th Avenue, Glendale, AZ 85308, USA
E-mail address: djenki@midwestern.edu

in podiatric medicine in 1974 quite in sync with not just the "jogging craze" but also the establishment of podiatric medicine as a major player in the world of sports medicine.

This article does not rehash the history of podiatric sports medicine per se, as an excellent treatise of this topic by Rich Bouché, DPM, a Past President of the American Academy of Podiatric Sports Medicine, is already available.[1] Instead, it evaluates the position of podiatrists as members of the sports medicine team, using the backdrop of history.

For those in podiatric medicine, the query as to the advantage and suitability of podiatrists on a multidisciplinary sports medicine team is self-evident, but what follows is an overview of why podiatrists are an invaluable part/component of a sports medicine team. This discussion is almost more to enlighten nonpodiatrists to the rationale of the inclusion of podiatrists on a sports medicine team.

HISTORY
Early Sports Medicine

Snook[2] presented an excellent historical review of Sports Medicine at large in the *American Journal of Sports Medicine* in 1984. Some of the interesting highlights, listed chronologically, are as follows:

1. The first recorded sports injury (an apparent hip dislocation in a wrestling match) is found in the Book of Genesis Holy Bible[3]
2. A compelling case is made by Anastasios and colleagues for why Herodicus (fifth century BC) should be considered the Father of Sports Medicine. Herodicus was in a unique position as he was not only a physician but also a physical educator. In that day, physicians did not typically have access to athletes but physical educators did. This access allowed Herodicus to use his methods with diet and exercise with top athletes of the day with reportedly excellent results. However, evidence is lacking that he was involved in care and treatment of injuries related to sports.[4]
3. Greek wrestler Milo of Croton (sixth century BC) was a renowned athlete and trainer. Although physicians of the day did attend to athletes if injured, trainers had the major role in managing nearly all the needs of athletes. There was certainly no physician dedicated to sport at that time. If the legendary tale that Milo's great strength came from daily hoisting of a newborn calf until it grew to a full-size bull is true, he would be the first to describe and participate in progressive resistance training.[2]
4. It seems Roman gladiators in the second century were the beneficiary of the first team doctor. The appointed physician was the medical superstar Claudius Galen. Snook,[5] whose publication is a major source for the history of sports medicine, argues that it is Galen who should be deemed the Father of Sports Medicine.
5. In sync with the significant dark period in science, sports medicine in the next number of centuries demonstrated little change or progress.[2]
6. In the United States, during the mid-1800s, Edward Hitchcock, MD, was becoming the foremost pioneer in the institution of Physical Education. Many consider Dr Hitchcock not only the Father of Physical Education but also the first sports medicine and team physician in the United States.[6]
7. In 1905, Dr Edward Nichols may have saved American football with his publications on morbidity and mortality and the resultant improvements through generated rule changes.[7]
8. Possibly the first team physician at the professional ranks was Dr Mal Stevens who in 1947 served as team physician to both the New York Yankees in baseball and the football New York Yankees of the All-American Conference.[2]

9. At the international level, sports medicine was the domain of physicians, whereas in the United States, it was that of nonphysicians (ie, athletic trainers, physical education instructors, physiologists). Accordingly, even treatment of athletic injuries in the United States near the turn of the century was provided by trainers and coaches. Early in the twentieth century, mainstream medicine left behind the concept of prevention and instead embraced the more exciting areas of surgery and pharmaceutical therapies.[1]

Consistent with this mind-set, some of the first US organizations for sports medicine were the American Association for Health, Physical Education and Recreation in the late 1800s, the National Athletic Trainers Association (NATA) in 1938, and the American College of Sports Medicine (ACSM) founded by Joseph Wolfe, a physiologist, in 1954.[1]

10. The first reported team of physicians present at the Olympics was in the 1968 Summer Games in Mexico City. Dr J. C. Kennedy and his team accompanied the team from Canada. Dr Kennedy then headed up the first official Olympic medical team in 1972 at Munich, Germany.[8]

Major Changes in the Mid-1970s

It is the author's perspective that before the 1970s sports medicine was little more than musculoskeletal injuries treated by orthopedic surgeons after they occurred; the concept of prevention and/or biomechanical interventions for sports-related injuries was unknown at that time, at least in prevailing medicine.

Podiatric Medicine's Entry into Sports Medicine

Podiatric medicine's mainstream prominence was due, in part, to the emergence of podiatric medicine as a major player in sports medicine; this coincided with the jogging boom in the mid-1970s, whereby running injuries were addressed not only preventively but also via biomechanical methods. The elaboration and success of this clinical approach as pointed out by George Sheehan, MD, in multiple venues including *Runner's World* put podiatric medicine on the map as Dr Sheehan identified podiatrists as, "The runner's doctor."

Other events during this time frame that vaulted podiatric medicine into the limelight of sports medicine was a collaboration of the University of California Medical Center and the California College of Podiatric Medicine. The conference "The Athlete's Dilemma: Overuse Syndrome of the Foot and Leg" held in San Francisco in 1973 resulted in a significant interdisciplinary meeting of minds. This conference, attended by the author, was the single most important event in the decision to become a podiatrist. To witness podiatrists highlighted with such specialists as renowned orthopedic surgeons as Richard Garrick and Stan James, as well as athletic trainers, chiropractors, and physical therapists, all collaborating, was an interdisciplinary paradise. Popular mainstream publications such as *"The Running Foot Doctor"* and *"The Foot Book"* by Steven Subotnick, DPM, and Harry Hlavac, DPM, respectively, were timely and further put podiatric medicine on the sports medicine playing field.

Birth of the American Academy of Podiatric Sports Medicine

In 1975, 13 podiatric physicians led by Robert Barnes, DPM, founded the American Academy of Podiatric Sports Medicine (AAPSM). The AAPSM, the representative body for podiatric physicians active in sports medicine, has played a major role in ensuring the inclusion of podiatric physicians in sports medicine activities and organizations. A detailed review of the history of podiatric sports medicine and the AAPSM has been compiled by Bouché[1] and is a major source for much of the historical content of this article.

Physician and Sports Medicine Round Table

With podiatrists still clamoring for legitimacy in the world of sports medicine, a pivotal article was published in *The Physician and Sports Medicine* in 1976 entitled "Foot Problems in Runners." This round table format showcased renowned orthopedists Sig Hansen, MD, and Stan James, MD, as well as podiatrists Steven Subotnick, DPM, and Stan Newell, DPM. Inclusion of podiatry on such an eminent stage was ultimately one more step to mainstream medicine's recognition of podiatric medicine's role in sports medicine.

Team Podiatrist at the Professional Ranks

A preeminent example of the podiatrist as a member of the sports medicine team may be attainment of the title Team Podiatrist for a professional sports team. Richard Gilbert, DPM, of San Diego, California, is credited with breaking through this barrier in the late 1970s.[1] Dr Gilbert served as team podiatrist for not only the National Football League San Diego Chargers but also the Major League Baseball Padres. Many podiatric physicians, too numerous to mention, have since become team podiatrists and consultants for professional and elite college sports teams.

Podiatric Medicine as a Member of the Olympic Medical Staff

Another participatory jewel on the Sports Medicine Team would be inclusion as a medical staff member at the Olympics Games. John Pagliano, DPM, a Past President of AAPSM as well as an elite runner, fought hard for the addition of podiatric physicians on the Olympic medical staff in the 1980s. His efforts were not successful but did come to fruition in 1996 when a team of podiatrists led by Past President of AAPSM Perry Julien, DPM, participated fully on the Olympic Medical Staff at the 1996 Olympic Summer Games in Atlanta (Bouché RT, unpublished data and personal communication, 2014). Lisa M. Schoene, DPM, ATC, podiatrist and athletic trainer, reported on her experiences as an official member of that medical staff in the Atlanta Olympic Summer Games of 1996.[9]

When the Olympic Winter Games were held in Salt Lake City, Utah, in 2002, AAPSM Past President Mike Lowe, DPM, led a team of podiatrists on the medical team (Bouché RT, unpublished data and personal communication, 2014).

CONCEPT OF A SPORTS MEDICINE TEAM
Sports Medicine Physician

When the concept of sports medicine (also referred to as sport and exercise medicine) began to evolve, it became more structured, whereupon many sports medicine entities such as a sports team organization appointed an individual as the team physician; this person was often a family physician who could not only attend to the day-to-day needs of the team's athletes such as routine physical examination and general medical issues but was also responsible for coordinating referrals to specialists for more sophisticated treatment (eg, anterior cruciate ligament [ACL] repair). In many current situations, professional sports teams have replaced the team doctor with a group of disparate specialties all with a keen contribution to the overall health and performance of the athlete. In most cases, the front-line care is provided by the training staff who also initiate referrals to needed specialists.

Concept of an Interdisciplinary Sports Medicine Setting

Multidisciplinary sports medicine clinic

Imagine a scenario whereby an athlete could attend a clinical venue populated with diverse health care specialists strongly interested in sports medicine. This athlete would not only receive multiple evaluations provided by this diverse group but could also benefit from the evaluators' common venue and their ability to discuss and consult each other with their respective findings.

In 1983, the author cofounded the Davis Area Sports Medicine Screening Clinic in the city of Davis, California, and although no treatment was provided, it consisted of the arrangement described earlier. Initially the clinic offered no-cost examinations of local athletes by orthopedists, physical therapists, and podiatrists, all of whom had a significant interest in sports medicine. During the next 5 years, the clinic expanded to also offer sports nutrition, sports psychology, sports vision, and sports dentistry as additional disciplines for the athlete being screened.

Although the athlete could elect to bypass some of the offered specialty evaluation stations at the clinic, most would take advantage of the diverse overview they could receive.

Of historical interest, the clinic's sport nutritionist was Liz Applegate, a graduate student at the University of California at Davis, who is now a nationally renowned expert on nutrition and fitness as well as a faculty member of the Nutrition Department and the Director of Sports Nutrition at the University of California, Davis.

This endeavor could not better exemplify the concept of an interdisciplinary practice. In many instances, an examination was done with several different clinicians jointly. A podiatric physician, orthopedic surgeon, and physical therapist may all look at a knee problem from a different perspective, and observing each other in a clinic such as this can provide huge educational opportunities for the clinicians as well as maximize the evaluative experience for the athlete. Most presenting complaints can benefit from these distinctive perspectives. Feedback from the athletes and the clinicians affirmed this sentiment.

The sports medicine team

A sports medicine team comprises disparate health professionals with unique knowledge, training, and skills who join together to provide an interdisciplinary assessment and/or treatment of an athlete.

This collaboration can be done separately or together to manage the athletes' needs, but as depicted earlier, significant advantages result from a common venue.

Team members invariably have a strong interest and/or experience in sports medicine and in many cases are former and/or current athletes themselves. Personal participation in sports by the clinician, especially if it is the same one as the athlete's, gives the clinician not only credibility but also empathy and understanding with regards to the athlete's issue for being seen. This concept of having "been in their shoes" cannot be overemphasized.

The athlete benefits from the varied backgrounds of the clinicians in that a given concern is addressed from multiple viewpoints based on diverse education, training, and experiences. In some cases, consultation between specialties can be done chair side with the patient, maximizing the athletes' overall experience and providing a comprehensive assessment.

Cons of an Interdisciplinary Sports Medicine Setting

A multidisciplinary sports medicine team is not without some downsides. A mixed specialty assessment was noted as a big plus for the athlete, but what about conflicts in opinion as to diagnosis or treatment? The very aspects thought to be advantages could result in friction especially in light of the individual's professional identity and associated training (eg, the typically greater biomechanical education seen in podiatric medicine). Preconceived bias and dearth of knowledge about the other specialty's education and training can feed into this dissention.

Issues of ego and "who's in charge?" could hamper a successful encounter, which also could be fed by individual specialists not informed as to knowledge and skills of others. Podiatric physicians, especially those trained pre-1980 are keenly aware of the struggle to inform not just other health care providers but the public at large as to the extensiveness of our education and training.

Some of the downsides are magnified if the members are not in direct communication. Disparate specialists involved in care of an athlete may not have knowledge of other consultant's involvement and rely on a trainers input only.

Members of a Sports Medicine Team and Their Contribution

The following list of professional participants in a sports medicine setting, although robust, is certainly not complete. In addition, not every specialty is represented in all sports medicine venues. This list could even include individuals not considered health care providers who nonetheless may play a triage role in the initial assessment and ultimate referral to a provider equipped to assist the athlete. An example of such an individual with whom many podiatric physicians are familiar and work closely with is the running shoe store retailer, often a front-line contact for runners with concerns or problems. These individuals are divided into 2 groups:

- Injury management
- Human performance

Injury Management
- Podiatric physicians
- Orthopedic physicians
- Physician assistants
- Nurse
- Dentists
- Physiatrist
- Chiropractors
- Physical therapists/trainers
- Massage therapists

Human Performance
- Strength and conditioning specialists
- Coaches
- Nutritionists
- Clinical psychologists
- Optometrists
- Exercise physiologists
- Biomechanists

The discipline of sports medicine has evolved greatly. It is no longer just a physician treating a sports injury but has become a multidisciplinary group of providers engaged in not only injury management but also injury prevention, as well as maximizing athletic performance through diet and training. This training has become more than just physical and may now include interventions such as mental conditioning (sports psychology) and vision (sports vision). For example, many athletes, especially at the elite level have found that an enhanced competitive edge may come from improvements in focus, relaxation, goal-setting, and anxiety reduction.

In perusing several existing interdisciplinary sports medicine organizations, it is not unusual to find the neurologist as a member given the heightened concerns about concussions.

The commonly thought of team members are, for the most part, clinical, those a patient may consult directly with to assess their concerns. Notwithstanding, behind the scenes, exercise physiologists and research biomechanists, to name two, make huge contributions to the practice of sports medicine.

WHAT DO PODIATRIC PHYSICIANS BRING TO THE TABLE?

As indicated by the title of this article, the underlying question that should be posed is: Why should podiatric physicians be included on a multidisciplinary sports medicine team? What can they offer that is unique to the team?

Lower Extremity Specialist

With a built-in focus on one area of the body, the lower extremities, no other specialty can claim such an immersion into just the lower extremity and in some cases the foot only. This focus results in markedly greater knowledge, skills, and experiences relevant to specialization in comparison to a clinician who may be responsible for multiple areas of the body such as an orthopedist.

Lower Extremity Multispecialist

Not all sports medicine afflictions are musculoskeletal in nature; hence, some lie outside the domain of orthopedics. The podiatrist has significant knowledge, training, and experience in addressing other systems such as dermatology, neurology, and vascular that typical orthopedists would not. For example, podiatrists often equal or exceed dermatologists when it comes to the evaluation and care of cutaneous afflictions of the lower extremity. Likewise, podiatric expertise in the realm of diabetes is unmatched by all except those specializing in diabetes. Like an orthopedic member of the team, and when considering the lower extremity only, the scope of practice is not restricted as to what treatment can be provided, although it may vary from state to state.

Biomechanics Expertise

Podiatric physicians bring to the table an unequaled biomechanics prowess. Podiatric medical students complete a curriculum that includes nearly 100 hours of didactic and laboratory training as well as numerous clinical electives of dedicated biomechanical training.[10] It is considered conventional wisdom that those podiatrists strongly involved in sports medicine tend to have a better-than-average interest and/or expertise in biomechanics.

There are some notable voices for podiatric biomechanics sounding the alarm that in the United States the realm of biomechanics seems to be trending away from podiatric medicine as physical therapists and others gain more training and knowledge and are now instituting an increased focus on biomechanical assessment and therapy in their practices. Perusing the literature gives an impression that podiatric medicine lags well behind international foot specialists, especially in Australia when it comes to publication of biomechanics studies. The emphasis on surgery in the US Colleges of Podiatric Medicine and during residency may be at fault. Past President of the

AAPSM Doug Riche, DPM, has been one such highly regarded expert in podiatric biomechanics who has been outspoken with regard to this trend (Bouché RT, unpublished data and personal communication, 2014).

This reported deemphasis on biomechanics education in the Colleges of Podiatric Medicine may be taking place at some colleges but is most definitely not the case at the Arizona School of Podiatric Medicine, which has maintained a strong emphasis of biomechanics in its curriculum.

Greater Toolbox

Most people who treat athletes or any patients would agree that instituting conservative care before recommending surgery is not only prudent but also imperative from a medicolegal and, in more and more cases, a reimbursement perspective. It can be argued that podiatric physicians possess a greater armamentarium for confronting injuries, especially with regards to the biomechanical therapies noted earlier. In countries where podiatrists are unable to perform surgery, use of nonsurgical options is maximized for lower extremity afflictions.

A case in point was in the early 1980s when the author was asked to consult on a college football running back with a pronounced tibial sesamoiditis. The solution, an orthotic made to offload the first metatarsal head and also incorporating a reverse Morton's extension, was hugely beneficial. Although the solution seemed routine for most podiatric physicians, it was lost on the physicians managing the team. Clearly at the time, podiatric physicians could bring to the table therapies that by all accounts were not readily appreciated or used in mainstream (primarily orthopedic) treatment.

HISTORY AND EXAMPLES OF PODIATRISTS AS MEMBERS OF THE SPORTS MEDICINE TEAM
"Sports Medicine" Podiatrists

The earliest podiatric practitioners of sports medicine were not labeled as such but were active in evaluating and treating injuries resulting from sports. Their inclusion in sports medicine circles was limited to membership in such organizations as ACSM and NATA.

Members of Multidisciplinary Clinical Sports Medicine Practices

As sports-minded health professionals organized the so-called sports medicine team that could offer a complete experience for athletes seeking care, many included podiatric medicine as a part of their team.

The Sports Medicine Clinic of Seattle, Washington, founded in 1963, touts itself as one of the first multidisciplinary sports medicine clinics in the country. The clinic is self-described as providing comprehensive sports medicine care under one roof. The list of team members denotes podiatrists as podiatric surgeons along with orthopedic surgeons.[11] This designation of equality is reflective of how far podiatric physicians have come.

Professional Sports Teams

Athletic trainers and/or physical therapists provide the lion's share of medical care to professional and college-level athletes. Physicians typically play a consulting role at this level, and as Bouché points out, podiatric sports medicine specialists, as a subspecialty, were well positioned to fit into this model.[1] This is not to say that professional or collegiate teams do not have team physicians; however, they just are not typically in the primary care role. It has been the author's experience that in nearly all cases of consultation at the collegiate and professional level, the request came from a trainer/physical therapist. Occasionally the request came from another specialist to provide a service they did not provide.

The good news is that many podiatric physicians have broken such an illustrious barrier in the care of athletes. The bad news is it would be logistically impossible to list all the podiatric physicians associated with professional and collegiate teams past and present.

Western States 100-Mile Endurance Run

The Western States 100-Mile Endurance Run (WS 100) was originally a horse race that commenced in 1955. The first "medical" stations were 3 veterinary stops set up for the horses. The WS 100 evolved into a foot race, with Gordy Ainsleigh the first to run the 100 miles in 1974. The first official race took place in 1977 and was termed the Western States 100-Mile Endurance Run. The 1978 event introduced organized medical checkpoints, which included podiatric medicine. This inclusion illustrated the significant role podiatrists were now playing in the care of runners.

At present, there are 10 major medical checkpoints including the finish line. The medical team is open to volunteers with medical skills (eg, DC, DDS, DO, DPM, EMT, LVN, MD, PA, Paramedic, RN). These important checkpoints are staffed by an impressively diverse group of health care practitioners. The author who has manned WS 100 aid stations at least 6 times during the 1980s believes the podiatric stations were the most important![12]

American College of Sports Medicine

ACSM is the largest sports medicine and exercise science organization in the world. With more than 50,000 members and certified professionals worldwide, ACSM is dedicated to advancing and integrating scientific research to provide educational and practical applications of exercise science and sports medicine. The ACSM mission is to advance and integrate scientific research to provide educational and practical applications of exercise science and sports medicine.[13]

The ACSM, as noted earlier, was founded in 1954. It could be considered the flagship of interdisciplinary sports medicine organizations. The melding of physical education, medicine, and physiology and their related investigators and clinicians is not unlike the scenario in ancient Greece as perceptively pointed out by Bouché.[1] The ACSM has welcomed podiatric physicians from its inception, long before podiatric sports medicine became a reality in the 1970s.

The relationship with the ACSM has grown stronger over the years, and although podiatrists had been members of the ACSM for quite some time, it was in 1977 that a dedicated track on podiatric sports medicine first took place at the annual ACSM conference.

In the mid-1990s, another barrier was overcome when AAPSM Past President Mark Julsrud, DPM, of Lacrosse, Wisconsin, became the first podiatrist to attain Fellowship status in the ACSM. As of this writing, 4 podiatric physicians are Fellows of the ACSM.

What once was simple inclusion in this reputable sports medicine organization became an opportunity to showcase the vast expertise held by podiatric sports medicine specialists. This was an excellent venue for networking with research biomechanists.

Joint Commission on Sports Medicine and Science

"To advance sports medicine by lacing together, through informal liaison and joint ventures, the nation's leading organizations in sports medicine and sports science" is the Mission Statement for the Joint Commission on Sports Medicine and Science (JCSMS).[14] This esteemed organization sought to bring together the most prominent and influential organizations in sports medicine. Only 32 such groups were invited, and the American Academy of Podiatric Sports Medicine was deemed one of the prime participants. As with the ACSM, podiatrists were positioned perfectly not only to network with diverse sports medicine specialties but also to showcase the significant knowledge and contributions podiatric physicians can make. This inclusion and opportunity to network at the annual JCSMS conference led to the subsequent affiliation between AAPSM and the Special Olympics, which occurred through a chance encounter when Rich Bouché, DPM, met Dr Mark Wagner, the Director, Special Olympics Health and Research Initiatives, and learned of Special Olympics' need for foot specialists to administer foot screenings for their athletes (Bouché RT, unpublished data and personal communication, 2014).

Special Olympics Healthy Athletes—Fit Feet

The Healthy Athletes initiative developed in 1997 provided vision, hearing, and dental screening; injury prevention clinics; and nutrition education to competing Special Olympics Athletes. In 2003, as a result of the chance meeting noted earlier and a great deal of hard work by AAPSM Past President Patrick Nunan, DPM, podiatric screenings (Fit Feet) were added to the Healthy Athletes Initiative. Fit Feet was the result of Special Olympics International's collaboration with the AAPSM and the International Federation of Podiatrists. To this date, more than 126,000 foot screenings have been performed.[15]

Fit Feet as part of a multidisciplinary screening event prominently placed podiatrists onto an international sports medicine team. Although large numbers of Fit Feet clinicians are podiatrists in the United States, this role is served by orthopedic surgeons in many other countries absent podiatrists. For those podiatrists who have participated at Special Olympics World Games such as the author who has been at 5, opportunities to interact and network with foot specialists from around the world are robust. Likewise, there is an astute appreciation of our training and knowledge.

Although the benefits to the Special Olympics athletes are self-evident, there have been substantial spin-offs such as podiatric student education, publications, and opportunities to evaluate conditions rarely found in the general population.

World Wide Web

In 1995, the first running injury Web site was developed by AAPSM Past President Stephen Pribut, DPM, further spreading the word about podiatric sports medicine to the masses via the World Wide Web.[16]

Benefits to Podiatric Medicine Education

Podiatric practitioners at large are not the only beneficiaries of podiatric medicine's membership on the sports medicine team. Students at the colleges of podiatric medicine can frequently participate under supervision in an array of major sports events. The WS 100, Special Olympics, and P. F. Chang's Rock 'n' Roll Arizona Marathon are just a few of the events at which the author has had the opportunity to supervise podiatric medical students. The interdisciplinary makeup of most of the medical teams often allows podiatric medical students to attend to medical issues as well as podiatric-related concerns.

SUMMARY

The history of sports medicine spans many centuries, and by comparison, podiatric medicine's involvement is in its infancy. It is remarkable how far a small profession has come in such a short period. What has been presented is an effort to explain how this happened against the backdrop of history.

As to how it happened, the reader should come away with the impression that, as with so many things, it has been a combination of many factors. Hard work, a passion for helping athletes, vocal advocates, and serendipity have all played a role in the dramatic ascension of podiatric medicine's place on the sports medicine stage.

REFERENCES

1. Bouché RT. Glancing back, striding ahead. The history of the American Academy of Podiatric Sports Medicine: part 1. J Am Podiatr Med Assoc 2003;93(4):315–20.
2. Snook GA. The history of sports medicine. Part I. Am J Sports Med 1984;12(4): 252–4.
3. Genesis 32:24, 25. Holy Bible, New International Version, NIV Copyright ©2011 by Biblica, Inc.
4. Georgoulis AD, Kiapidou IS, Velogianni L. Herodicus, the Father of Sports Medicine. Knee Surg Sports Traumatol Arthrosc 2007;15:315–8.
5. Snook GA. The Father of Sports Medicine (Galen). Am J Sports Med 1978;6(3): 128–31.
6. Welch JE. Pioneering in health education and services at Amherst College. J Am Coll Health 1982;30(6):289–95.
7. Nichols EH, Richardson FL. Football injuries of the Harvard squad for three years under the revised rules. 1909. Clin Orthop Relat Res 2003;(409):3–10.
8. Altius Directory. Available at: http://www.altiusdirectory.com/Sports/sports-medicine.html. Accessed September 15, 2014.
9. Sports Medicine Associates Web page. Available at: http://drschoene.com/press-room/featured-magazine-newspaper-articles/working-as-a-sports-medicine-podiatrist-at-the-olympics. Accessed September 15, 2014.
10. Midwestern University Course Catalog 2014-2015. Arizona School of Podiatric Medicine; 153–162.
11. The Sports Medicine Clinic Web Page. Available at: http://www.thesports medicineclinic.com/services/default.asp. Accessed September 16, 2014.
12. Western States 100-Mile Endurance Run Web Site. http://www.wser.org/how-it-all-began/. Accessed September 16, 2014.
13. American College of Sports Medicine Web Site. Available at: http://acsm.org/. Accessed September 17, 2014.
14. Web site for the Joint Commission on Sports Medicine & Science. Available at: http://jcsmsonline.org/. Accessed September 17, 2014.
15. Special Olympics Web site. Available at: http://www.specialolympics.org/default. aspx. Accessed September 17, 2014.
16. Dr Pribut's Running Injuries Page Web site. Available at: http://www.drpribut.com/sports/sportframe.html. Accessed September 17, 2014.

Two Emerging Technologies for Achilles Tendinopathy and Plantar Fasciopathy

Paul R. Langer, DPM, ABPM, FAAPSM*

KEYWORDS

- Achilles tendinopathy • Plantar fasciitis • Extracorporeal shock wave therapy
- Percutaneous tenotomy • Percutaneous fasciotomy

KEY POINTS

- Some overuse musculoskeletal injuries can be resistant to standard therapies. Alternative therapies may be considered earlier in the continuum of care and before surgical options are pursued.
- Extracorporeal shock wave therapy is becoming a more commonly used treatment modality in sports medicine and provides a noninvasive treatment option for tendon and fascia injuries.
- Ultrasound-guided percutaneous tenotomy/fasciotomy is a newer, minimally invasive technology that provides additional treatment options that may be considered before more invasive surgical interventions.

By some estimates 10% to 25% of individuals affected by Achilles tendinopathy and plantar fasciitis fail conservative treatment.[1–3] For those individuals who fail nonoperative modalities, operative intervention is often the next option. Recently, 2 other treatment options have shown potential as viable options for treatment of these conditions before surgery.

EXTRACORPOREAL SHOCK WAVE THERAPY

The use of acoustic energy in the form of unique sets of "high-energy" acoustic pressure waves or sound waves to treat musculoskeletal injuries has been around for approximately 30 years and the volume of research on effect, potential benefit, and

Disclosures: None.
Department of Family Practice, University of Minnesota Medical School, Minneapolis, Minnesota
* Corresponding author.
E-mail address: paullanger@tcomn.com

Clin Podiatr Med Surg 32 (2015) 183–193
http://dx.doi.org/10.1016/j.cpm.2014.11.002   podiatric.theclinics.com
0891-8422/15/$ – see front matter © 2015 Elsevier Inc. All rights reserved.

mechanism of action continues to grow. Shock wave therapy (SWT) is a relatively new technology that has become increasingly popular as a treatment for musculoskeletal conditions, in part because it is noninvasive and clinically and economically effective. It also allows athletes to remain active during the treatment process. SWT is approved and/or cleared by the US Food and Drug Administration for treatment of musculoskeletal pain, plantar fasciitis, and lateral epicondylitis, and has been used for other off-label indications, including tendonopathies and other musculoskeletal conditions.[4] Overall, research is mixed in terms of the effectiveness of SWT.[4–7] A significant limitation to drawing definitive conclusions about the effectiveness of SWT is the variability in study design and methods, which makes it difficult to pools results. More research needs to be done to better elucidate effectiveness, optimal methodologies, adjunctive treatments, and posttreatment protocols.

Background and Technology

In the 1980s, shock waves began to be used to treat kidney stones.[8] The research on animals that preceded this clinical use suggested that there were also potentially beneficial effects on musculoskeletal structures. Subsequent research on the effects on bone, cartilage, muscle, tendon and ligaments eventually led to other clinical applications and SWT has become increasingly popular as a treatment modality. SWT is often called extracorporeal SWT.

Therapeutic shock waves are unique sets of acoustic pressure waves directed through a medium. They are typically classified as either focused or unfocused. Focused waves were used more commonly in the earlier days of clinical application, but recently unfocussed (or, as they are more commonly called, "radial") pressure waves are used with increasing frequency. Radial pressure waves are used increasingly more often because they can be applied without local anesthesia and have the potential to be less injurious. In addition, improved technology makes the machines less costly to own and operate, and more convenient to use in clinical settings.[3,9] Multiple investigators have concluded that no evidence clearly favors either focused or radial shock wave therapy.[4,10] Other authors have shown that extracorporeal SWT delivered without local anesthesia was more effective compared with delivery under local anesthesia.[11,12] Because radial SWT (RSWT) is being used more commonly in clinical settings and can be delivered without local anesthesia, it is the focus of this review.

Ogden and colleagues[13] described therapeutic shock wave as a "controlled explosion" that will be reflected, refracted, transmitted, and dissipated as it travels through tissue. As it travels, a pressure phase is followed by a low-pressure or tensile phase, and then cavitation follows. Any change in tissue type presents a boundary, and it is at these boundaries or tissue interfaces where the biological effects of cavitation occur.[14,15] Structures like cartilage and bone reflect the energy of the wave, whereas structures with high collagen content, such as tendon, ligament, and joint capsule, tend to absorb the wave.[16,17]

The shock wave can be generated in a number of different ways, but the most commonly used and clinically validated method for RSWT is pneumatic. The energy content of the pressure wave can be varied depending on the selected settings and equipment; the propagation of the wave will vary with tissue type. With radial acoustic pressure waves, the skin is subjected to the greatest concentration of energy; as the wave travels through other tissues, a steep drop off of energy occurs. Structures that are close to the skin surface are especially impacted by SWT (**Fig. 1**).[4]

The acoustic pressure wave can be manipulated in a number of ways, one of which is by varying the amount of energy per unit area per pulse. This is known as the energy

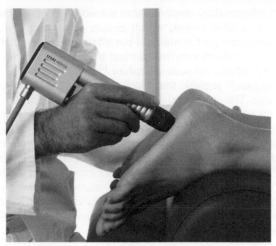

Fig. 1. Radial wave therapy machine with hand piece positioned to treat plantar fasciitis. (*Courtesy of* CuraMedix LLC, Lincoln, RI; with permission.)

flux density (EFD) and is measured in mJ/mm^2. The safe, effective range of EFD is approximately between 0.14 and 0.5 mJ/mm^2.[18–20] The pulses per second can be adjusted as well and are measured in Hertz (Hz). The total number of shocks delivered per treatment session typically varies from 500 to 3000, depending on the tissue being treated, depth of tissue penetration requirements, clinical judgment, research, and manufacturer recommendations. Finally, the number of treatments and interval between treatments has not been standardized, but 3 to 5 weekly treatments are a common protocol seen for Achilles tendinopathy and plantar fasciitis.

There have not been many studies or consistent recommendations on the proper "dose" of shock waves for specific pathologies. This is an area that clearly needs more study, not only to improve understanding of the technology, but also to better track outcomes. Tam and associates[21] proposed calculating a total energy dose by multiplying the EFD by the number of shocks to quantify treatment dose and provide objective data for outcomes studies.

Rompe[22] stated that level I therapeutic studies have provided evidence for plantar fasciitis treatment benefits utilizing the following protocol:

1. Application of 1500 to 2000 shocks at an EFD 0.08 to 0.15 mJ/mm^2;
2. Application to site of maximal discomfort via patient guidance;
3. No local anesthesia;
4. Three to 4 applications spaced at 1 week between applications; and
5. At least 3 months of follow-up after the last treatment.

Biologic Effects

Research is starting to elucidate some of the mechanisms for how shock waves promote tissue repair. There have been immediate, short-term, and extended effects reported, but the mechanism for these effects remain poorly understood. The primary mechanisms of healing response most often cited in the literature are ones of an initial inflammatory response followed by neovascularization. Saxena and colleagues[23] described RSWT as creating "a controlled, microtrauma to local affected tissue to stimulate a healing response and micro-vascularization." The initial microtrauma causes a transient inflammatory response that subsides in approximately 1 week and is followed by a remodeling phase, which occurs at around 3 weeks after treatment.[13,14] Some subjects report immediate but often temporary analgesia after treatment. These analgesic effects may be derived from hyperstimulation, depletion of substance P, or other effects on pain receptors.[19,24,25]

Weihs and colleagues[26] showed that SWT enhances cell proliferation in vitro and wound healing in vivo. They identified adenosine triphosphate as a trigger of a chemical cascade that then leads to a healing response via purinergic signaling and, eventually, increased collagen synthesis.[27] Neovascularization effects have been shown through angiogenesis via cellular mediators, such as vascular endothelial growth factor, as well as enhanced expression of other proangiogenic cells, including cytokines and fibroblasts.[28-31] The neovascularization effect increased in the first 8 weeks and was still present at 12 weeks in a rat tendon study reported by Takahashi and co-workers in 2003.[32] Because neovascularization and collagen synthesis are slower to occur events in healing, it is speculated that maximum benefit of RSWT may be 90 to 120 days, or later, after treatment.

Podiatric Indications

Two common conditions treated by podiatric physicians that can be refractory to conventional treatment are Achilles tendinopathy and plantar fasciopathy. Patients who have failed conventional therapies are often faced with the prospects of living with their condition, considering operative interventions, or considering newer and alternative therapies or treatments. The bulk of the literature on lower extremity conditions and RSWT is found for these 2 conditions. Potential benefits are best when combining SWT with tissue-specific stretching and strengthening exercises, as well as tissue loading changes.[5,6,33,34]

Achilles tendinopathy

Rasmussen and colleagues,[35] in a randomized, double-blinded, placebo-controlled trial in 2008 found improved function scores in subjects treated with extracorporeal SWT, stretching, and eccentric exercises versus sham treatment, stretching, and eccentric exercises at 8 and 12 weeks after treatment. However, the test subjects had no significant change in pain scores. The combination of radial shock waves and eccentric loading tended to provide faster symptom relief compared with treatment alone, but no difference in outcome was found after 1 year in a study by Rompe and associates in 2009.[6] In a review of the literature, Foldager and colleagues[4] found that, for both insertional and noninsertional Achilles tendinopathy, shock wave therapy showed a significant benefit. However, Magnussen and co-workers,[36] in a systematic review, concluded that more research needed to be done before drawing conclusions. Saxena and colleagues,[37] in a prospective study on 74 tendons, showed reduced pain and improved function in 78% of subjects 1 year after treatment with RSWT. They noted no adverse events and athletic individuals were able to continue their activity.

Plantar fasciitis

Sems and associates[38] review from 2006 concluded that there was a "preponderance" of the evidence to support the use of shock wave for refractory plantar fasciitis and noted that directing the shock wave at the calcaneal spur or maximal area of pain provided the most favorable results.

Other studies have shown benefits of shock wave in treating plantar fasciitis as well. Gerdesmeyer and colleagues,[39] in a randomized, double-blinded study with 115 patients, reported significantly reduced pain scores compared with untreated control group. They treated in 3 sessions of 2000 shocks each spaced weekly, at an EFD of 0.16 mJ/mm^2, and found significant pain reduction at 12 weeks compared with un-treated control group. Ibrahim and colleagues[40] in 2010 achieved reduced pain scores on a visual analog scale in 50 patients treated with 2 treatments of 2000 pulses spaced 1 week apart versus a placebo treatment group.

Two small studies failed to show significant benefit of SWT. Mark's study of 25 sub-jects failed to show a benefit of 3 treatments spaced 3 days apart using 500 to 2000 shocks.[41] Greve and colleagues[42] found benefit of SWT, but it was not superior to plantar fascia stretching exercises in a study with 36 subjects. Hsu and associates[43] found reduced pain and improved gait parameters in 12 patients after 3 weekly treat-ments of SWT.

Adverse Effects

The most common side effects reported are minor, such as petechial bleeding, swelling, and discomfort during treatment.[4,9,12,22,23,34] A case report described an Achilles tendon rupture after a single shock wave treatment. However, the patient had also undergone multiple other treatments including calcaneal exostectomy and cortisone injections.[44]

Summary

Despite mixed results in the literature, RSWT may be a viable treatment option after other treatments have failed and before considering surgical intervention for Achilles tendinopathy and plantar fasciitis. The literature is more conclusive in the benefits for plantar fasciitis. Although more research needs to be done, shock wave therapy does show potential to be a safe and effective adjunct treatment option for refractory conditions.

PERCUTANEOUS ULTRASONIC FASCIOTOMY FOR PLANTAR FASCIOSIS

Recently, percutaneous ultrasonic tenotomy and fasciotomy have become available to treat chronic tendon disease and plantar fasciosis.[45–48] This minimally invasive technique is based on the physical principles of phacoemulsification, whereby ultra-sonic energy is utilized to precisely emulsify and remove tissue in the vicinity of a work-ing tip that oscillates at high frequencies.[45,49] Although phacoemulsification was originally popularized to remove cataracts, the technology has been further developed to treat tendon and fascial disease percutaneously using a hand piece and portable console (Tenex Health, Inc., Lake Forrest, CA, USA).[45,49]

Technology and Instruments

The hand piece contains an 18-gauge, inner, stainless steel tube connected to a series of piezoelectric crystals electronically driven at high frequencies to produce low-amplitude oscillations in the working tip (Fig. 2). The central lumen of this tube is attached to a suction system within the console that aspirates lavage fluid and tissue debris into a collection bag. The inner tube is surrounded by an outer plastic tube that is slightly recessed, thus exposing only a small portion of the working tip. Pressurized lavage fluid emerges between the outer plastic tube and the stainless steel inner tube, cooling the working tip and providing fluid for lavage and debris removal. The working tip is controlled by a foot pedal that activates the ultrasonic energy. When activated, the working tip oscillates while pressurized fluid emerges into the working field and is aspirated through the central lumen of the inner tube. Tissue within 1 mm of the work-ing tip is emulsified and aspirated via the process of cavitation.

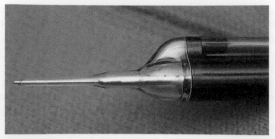

Fig. 2. The TX1 working tip, demonstrating the distal end of the hand piece and the working tip. Note the plastic outer tube, through which the 18-gauge, stainless steel inner tube protrudes slightly. When the piezoelectric crystals in the hand piece are activated by the foot pedal, the inner tube vibrates with high-frequency, low-amplitude oscillations, emulsifying tissue within 1 mm of the tip. Pressurized fluid flows into the working area between the plastic outer tube and stainless steel inner tube, and is removed via a vacuum suction through the lumen of the inner stainless steel tube. The fluid inflow–outflow is continuous during working tip activating, cooling the tip and removing emulsified tissue, which is collected in a bag attached to the TX1 desktop console (not shown).

Percutaneous ultrasonic fasciotomy can be used to treat chronic plantar fasciosis under ultrasound guidance.[50] The most common indication is chronic, refractory plantar fasciosis unresponsive to standard treatments and accompanied by structural changes as identified on ultrasonography or MRI. The exact mechanism of action has not been determined precisely, but percutaneous ultrasonic fasciotomy likely works primarily by removing the pathologic tissue associated with pain and consequently facilitating a healing response.[45] Koh and colleagues[47] reported improvements in the ultrasonographic appearance of the common extensor tendon after successful treatment of lateral elbow tendinopathy with percutaneous ultrasonic tenotomy. Current investigations are ongoing to determine the histologic changes over time after percutaneous ultrasonic tenotomy.

Treating Plantar Fasciopathy

To perform percutaneous ultrasonic fasciotomy, the plantar fascia is first examined using standard ultrasonographic techniques.[48,50] Plantar fasciosis manifests as diffuse or focal thickening, heterogeneity, and hypoechogenicity (ie, dark) of the plantar fascia, typically affecting the central cord (**Fig. 3**).[48,51] In some cases, these ultrasonographic findings may be accompanied by focal, hypoechoic–anechoic regions representing partial thickness tearing, Doppler flow consistent with neovascularization, and/or cortical irregularities, including plantar calcaneal spurs.[49] The affected region of the plantar fascia is identified and the skin marked with an indelible ink marker.

The patient is typically placed prone or in a lateral decubitus position for a medial to lateral approach, short axis to the plantar fascia. However, a long axis approach to the plantar fascia is possible.[48,50] The area is prepared in the usual sterile fashion and the use of appropriate draping, sterile ultrasound transducer covers and sterile ultrasound gel can ensure sterile working conditions throughout the procedure. The plantar fascia is identified in the short axis and local anesthesia is obtained using 1% lidocaine and a ultrasonographically guided, in-plane, medial to lateral approach with a 25-gauge needle or equivalent (an ultrasound-guided tibial nerve block may be performed as an alternative for anesthesia).[48,51] Approximately 4 to 8 mL of lidocaine are injected into the skin, subcutaneous tissue, fat pad, and superficial portions of the plantar

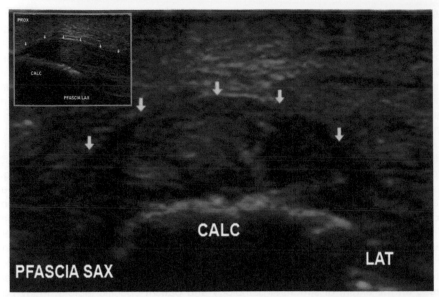

Fig. 3. Correlative short axis ultrasound view of a thickened, heterogenous, hypoechoic plantar fascia (PFASCIA) typical of chronic plantar fasciosis. *Top,* Plantar/superficial; *bottom,* dorsal/deep; *left,* medial; *right,* lateral (LAT). Arrows identify superficial portion of plantar fascia. Inset shows correlative long axis (LAX) view, proximal to the left. CALC, calcaneus.

fascia at the anticipated point of entry. Thereafter, a small stab incision is completed (blade oriented parallel to the plantar aspect of the foot) using a #11 scalpel blade to creating a 2- to 3-mm skin incision. The blade is advanced toward the plantar fascia using direct ultrasound guidance. After this, the TX1 tip is advanced using a similar sonographically guided, in plane, medial to lateral approach, until it contacts the medial aspect of the affected portion of the plantar fascia (**Fig. 4**). Some users prefer to precede TX1 placement by passage of a 14-gauge needle to create a wider channel for the TX1 tip. Once the TX1 tip is placed adjacent to the plantar fascia, the working tip is activated via the foot pedal. The operator gently moves the TX1 tip into the plantar

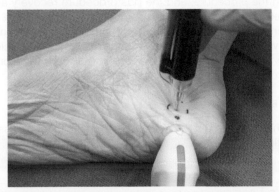

Fig. 4. After delivery of local anesthesia as described in the text, a small stab incision is created with a #11 scalpel blade to create a passage to advance the TX1 working tip to the plantar fascia under direct ultrasound guidance. *Left,* distal (toes); *right,* proximal (heel).

fascia using direct ultrasound guidance. As the tip enters the fascia, the fascia is cut via phacoemulsification and the debris and inflow fluid removed via the hand piece outflow and transferred into the collection bag on the console.[45,50] During the fasciotomy and debridement process, the operator moves the working tip in low-amplitude, back-and-forth motions while its position is monitored using orthogonal ultrasound imaging.[45–47,50] Typically, 4- to 5-second pulses of energy are used, with a total energy time of 30 seconds to 2 minutes, depending on the size of the treated region. Using ultrasound imaging, all affected areas are treated as dictated by the clinical scenario.

At the completion of treatment, the TX1 tip is removed, the wound dressed with adhesive strips, a pressure gauze bandage and sterile occlusive dressing, and postprocedural instructions are reviewed with the patient.[45,50] Edema control, icing, range of motion, and gentle stretching are recommended for all patients immediately after the procedure until the initial follow-up. Some patients may benefit from a period of modified weight bearing in a walking boot and/or crutches as dictated by the extent of treated pathology and individual clinician's preference.[50] Over-the-counter analgesic and anti-inflammatory medications can be taken as necessary; prescription-strength medications are not often required. Patients are typically seen 2 to 4 weeks after the procedure, at which time rehabilitation and return to activities is individualized based on the extent of structural pathology and patient-specific factors. Many patients may return to running 6 to 8 weeks after the procedure, although the recovery course can be highly variable.[50] Of note, as is the case for some minimally invasive procedures, many patients experience early pain relief before adequate tissue healing, placing them at risk to overstress the healing tissues early in the rehabilitation process. Patients should be counseled accordingly.

Percutaneous ultrasonic tenotomy and fasciotomy is a well-tolerated, minimally invasive outpatient procedure that seems to be both safe and effective when applied to a variety of tendons throughout the body, as well as the plantar fascia.[45–47,50] Two prospective case series including a total of 39 patients have documented satisfactory results in more than 80% of patients with chronic, refractory elbow tendinosis at 1 year after treatment.[47,48] The total energy time for patients in these series was generally less than 60 seconds, with total treatment times of approximately 15 minutes, including preparation and skin marking.[46,47] No complications were reported in either series.[46,47] With respect to the plantar fascia, the total procedure time is also typically less than 15 minutes, patients typically require no more than 10 mL of 1% lidocaine for anesthesia during the procedure, and the postprocedure recovery and rehabilitation are uncomplicated. Patel and colleagues[48] recently reported 100% satisfactory results at 2 years among 12 patients (13 feet) with greater than 12 months of refractory plantar fasciosis who were treated with percutaneous ultrasonic fasciotomy. Percutaneous ultrasonic fasciotomy seems to warrant further consideration as a definitive treatment for chronic, refractory plantar fasciosis.

ACKNOWLEDGMENTS

The author of this article would like to thank Dr. Jay Smith for his assistance in preparation of this article.

REFERENCES

1. Alfredson H, Pietilä T, Jonsson P, et al. Heavy-load eccentric calf muscle training for the treatment of chronic Achilles tendinosis. Am J Sports Med 1998;26(3): 360–6.

2. Davis PF, Severud E, Baxter DE. Painful heel syndrome: results of non-operative treatment. Foot Ankle Int 1994;15(10):531–5, 4.

3. Malay DS. Plantar fasciitis and heel spur syndrome: a retrospective analysis. In: Vickers NS, editor. Reconstructive surgery of the foot and leg: update '96. Tucker (GA): Podiatry Institute Publishing; 1996. p. 39–43.

4. Foldager CB, Kearney C, Spector M. Clinical application of extracorporeal shock wave therapy in orthopedics: focused versus unfocused shock waves. Ultrasound Med Biol 2012;38(10):1673–80.

5. van der Worp H, van den Akker-Scheek I, van Schie H, et al. ESWT for tendinopathy: technology and clinical implications. Knee Surg Sports Traumatol Arthrosc 2013;21(6):1451–8.

6. Rompe JD, Furia J, Maffulli N. Eccentric loading versus eccentric loading plus shock-wave treatment for midportion Achilles tendinopathy: a randomized controlled trial. Am J Sports Med 2009;37:463–70.

7. Chung B, Wiley JP. Extracorporeal shockwave therapy—a review. Sports Med 2002;32:851–65.

8. Chaussy C, Schuller J, Schmiedt E, et al. Extracorporeal shock-wave lithotripsy (ESWL) for treatment of urolithiasis. Urology 1984;23:59–66.

9. Watson T. Shock wave therapy. Available at: www.electrotherapy.org. Accessed September 12, 2014.

10. van der Worp H, Zwerver J, Hamstra M, et al. No difference in effectiveness between focused and radial shockwave therapy for treating patellar tendinopathy: a randomized controlled trial. Knee Surg Sports Traumatol Arthrosc 2014;22(9):2026–32.

11. Labek G, Auersperg V, Ziernhold M, et al. Influence of local anesthesia and energy level on the clinical outcome of extracorporeal shock wave-treatment of chronic plantar fasciitis—a prospective randomized clinical trial. Z Orthop Ihre Grenzgeb 2005;143:240–6.

12. Rompe JD, Meurer A, Nafe B, et al. Repetitive low-energy shock wave application without local anesthesia is more efficient than repetitive low-energy shock wave application with local anesthesia in the treatment of chronic plantar fasciitis. J Orthop Res 2005;23:931–41.

13. Ogden JA, Alvarez RG, Levitt R, et al. Shock wave therapy (orthotripsy (R)) in musculoskeletal disorders. Clin Orthop Relat Res 2001;(387):22–40.

14. Ogden JA, Toth-Kischkat A, Schultheiss R. Principles of shock wave therapy. Clin Orthop Relat Res 2001;(387):8–17.

15. Kearney CJ, Lee JY, Padera RF, et al. Extracorporeal shock wave-induced proliferation of periosteal cells. J Orthop Res 2011;29:1536–43.

16. Watson T. Ultrasound in contemporary physiotherapy practice. Ultrasonics 2008; 48(4):321–9.

17. Watson T, Young S. Therapeutic ultrasound. In: Watson T, editor. Electrotherapy: evidence based practice. Edinburgh (Scotland): Churchill-Livingstone, Elsevier; 2008.

18. Maier M, Tischer T, Milz S, et al. Dose-related effects of extracorporeal shock waves on rabbit quadriceps tendon integrity. Arch Orthop Trauma Surg 2002; 122:436–41.

19. Rompe JD, Kirkpatrick CJ, Kullmer K, et al. Dose-related effects of shock waves on rabbit tendon Achilles—A sonographic and histological study. J Bone Joint Surg Br 1998;80:546–52.

20. Bosch G, de Mos M, van Binsbergen R, et al. The effect of focused extracorporeal shock wave therapy on collagen matrix and gene expression in normal tendons and ligaments. Equine Vet J 2009;41:335–41.

21. Tam KF, Cheung WH, Lee KM, et al. Delayed stimulatory effect of low-intensity shockwaves on human periosteal cells. Clin Orthop Relat Res 2005;438:260–5.
22. Rompe JD. Letter to the editor: shock wave therapy for chronic Achilles tendon pain: a randomized placebo-controlled trial. Clin Orthop Relat Res 2006;445: 276–7.
23. Saxena A, Fournier M, Gerdesmeyer L, et al. Comparison between extracorporeal shockwave therapy, placebo ESWT and endoscopic plantar fasciotomy for the treatment of chronic plantar heel pain in the athlete. Muscles Ligaments Tendons J 2013;2(4):312–6.
24. Mittermayr R, Hartinger J, Antonic V, et al. Extracorporeal shock wave therapy (ESWT) minimizes ischemic tissue necrosis irrespective of application time and promotes tissue revascularization by stimulating angiogenesis. Ann Surg 2011; 253:1024–32.
25. Hausdorf J, Lemmens MA, Kaplan S, et al. Extracorporeal shockwave application to the distal femur of rabbits diminishes the number of neurons immunoreactive for substance P in dorsal root ganglia L5. Brain Res 2008;1207:96–101.
26. Weihs AM, Fuchs C, Teuschl AH, et al. Shockwave treatment enhances cell proliferation and improves wound healing by ATP release coupled extracellular signal-regulated kinase (ERK) activation. J Biol Chem 2014;289(39):27090–104. http://dx.doi.org/10.1074/jbc.M114.580936.
27. Vetrano M, d'Alessandro F, Torrisi MR, et al. Extracorporeal shock wave therapy promotes cell proliferation and collagen synthesis of primary cultured human tenocytes. Knee Surg Sports Traumatol Arthrosc 2011;19:2159–68.
28. Hayashi D, Kawakami K, Ito K, et al. Low-energy extracorporeal shock wave therapy enhances skin wound healing in diabetic mice: a critical role of endothelial nitric oxide synthase. Wound Repair Regen 2012;20:887–95.
29. Kuo YR, Wang CT, Wang FS, et al. Extracorporeal shock-wave therapy enhanced wound healing via increasing topical blood perfusion and tissue regeneration in a rat model of STZ-induced diabetes. Wound Repair Regen 2009;17:522–30.
30. Dumfarth J, Zimpfer D, Vogele-Kadletz M, et al. Prophylactic low-energy shock wave therapy improves wound healing after vein harvesting for coronary artery bypass graft surgery: a prospective, randomized trial. Ann Thorac Surg 2008; 86:1909–13.
31. Yan X, Zeng B, Chai Y, et al. Improvement of blood flow, expression of nitric oxide, and vascular endothelial growth factor by low-energy shockwave therapy in random-pattern skin flap model. Ann Plast Surg 2008;61:646–53.
32. Takahashi N, Wada Y, Ohtoori S, et al. Application of shock waves to rat skin decreases calcitonin gene-related peptide immunoreactivity in dorsal root ganglion neurons. Neuroscience 2003;107:81–4.
33. Peers KH. Extracorporeal shock wave therapy in chronic Achilles and patellar tendinopathy [Dissertation or thesis]. KU Leuven; 2003 (ISBN: 9058673049).
34. Kountouris A, Cook J. Rehabilitation of Achilles and patellar tendinopathies. Best Pract Res Clin Rheumatol 2007;21:295–316.
35. Rasmussen S, Christensen M, Mathiesen I, et al. Shockwave therapy for chronic Achilles tendinopathy: a double-blind, randomized clinical trial of efficacy. Acta Orthop 2008;79(2):249–56.
36. Magnussen RA, Dunn WR, Thomson AB. Nonoperative treatment of midportion Achilles tendinopathy: a systematic review. Clin J Sport Med 2009;19:54–64.
37. Saxena A, Ramdath S, O'Halloran P, et al. Extra-corporeal pulsed-activated therapy ("EPAT" sound wave) for Achilles tendinopathy: a prospective study. J Foot Ankle Surg 2011;50(3):315–9.

38. Sems A, Dimeff R, Iannotti JP. Extracorporeal shock wave therapy in the treatment of chronic tendinopathies. J Am Acad Orthop Surg 2006;14(4):195–204.
39. Gerdesmeyer L, Frey C, Vester J, et al. Radial extracorporeal shock wave therapy is safe and effective in the treatment of chronic recalcitrant plantar fasciitis results of a confirmatory randomized placebo- controlled multicenter study. Am J Sports Med 2008;36:2100–9.
40. Ibrahim MI, Donatelli RA, Schmitz C, et al. Chronic plantar fasciitis treated with two sessions of radial extracorporeal shock wave therapy. Foot Ankle Int 2010; 31:391–7.
41. Marks W, Jackiewicz A, Witkowski Z, et al. Extracorporeal shock-wave therapy (ESWT) with a new-generation pneumatic device in the treatment of heel pain. A double blind randomised controlled trial. Acta Orthop Belg 2008;74:98–101.
42. Greve JM, Grecco MV, Santos-Silva PR. Comparison of radial shockwaves and conventional physiotherapy for treating plantar fasciitis. Clinics (Sao Paulo) 2009;64:97–103.
43. Hsu WH, Lai LJ, Chang HY, et al. Effect of shockwave therapy on plantar fascio-pathy A biomechanical prospective. Bone Joint J 2013;95-B(8):1088–93.
44. Lin TC, Lin CY, Chou CL, et al. Achilles tendon tear following shock wave therapy for calcific tendinopathy of the Achilles tendon: a case report. Phys Ther Sport 2012;13(3):189–92.
45. Barnes DE. Ultrasonic energy in tendon treatment. Op Tech Orthopaed 2013;23: 78–83.
46. Barnes DE, Beckley JM, Smith J. Percutaneous ultrasonic tenotomy for chronic elbow tendinosis: a prospective study. J Shoulder Elbow Surg 2014;24:67–73.
47. Koh JS, Mohan PC, Howe TS, et al. Fasciotomy and surgical tenotomy for recal-citrant lateral elbow tendinopathy. Early clinical experience with a novel device for minimally invasive percutaneous microresection. Am J Sports Med 2013;41: 636–44.
48. Patel MM. A novel treatment method for refractory plantar fasciitis. Am J Orthop, in press.
49. Packer M, Fishkind WJ, Fine H, et al. The physics of phaco: a review. J Cataract Refract Surg 2005;31:424–31.
50. Smith J, Finnoff JT. Diagnosis and interventional musculoskeletal ultrasound. Part 1. Fundamentals. PM R 2009;1:64–75.
51. Smith J, Finnoff JT. Diagnosis and interventional musculoskeletal ultrasound. Part 2. Clinical applications. PM&R 2009;1:162–77.

Return to Play After an Ankle Sprain

Guidelines for the Podiatric Physician

Douglas H. Richie, DPM, FACFAS, FAAPSM*, Faye E. Izadi, DPM

KEYWORDS

- Ankle sprain • Return to play • Return to sport • Chronic ankle instability
- Functional ankle testing • Athlete

KEY POINTS

- The ankle sprain is the most common injury in sport and has a high incidence of long-term disability. Athletes who develop permanent sequelae from an ankle sprain may have returned to sport before they had time to fully recover and heal their injury.
- An individualized rehabilitation program that follows evidence-based protocols is critical to the recovery from an ankle sprain. The mechanical and functional components of chronic ankle instability (CAI) are preventable through proper rehabilitation.
- There are key guidelines that a podiatric physician can follow to help in determining when an athlete is ready to return to sport after an injury. Patient-based questionnaires in addition to functional performance testing can be used to critically assess the status of ankle function before returning an athlete to play.
- Once an athlete is cleared to return to sport, prophylactic measures to prevent reinjury to the ankle should be implemented.

INTRODUCTION

The ankle sprain is the most common injury in sport, comprising up to 45% of all injuries.[1] Ankle sprains account for 10% of all visits to hospital emergency rooms, and their incidence has been on a steady increase during the past 30 years because of greater overall participation in recreational sports in the United States.[2,3] Podiatric physicians commonly encounter patients who are at some stage of recovery from an acute ankle sprain.[4]

Regardless of whether treatment is sought or which medical specialty provides the treatment, it is well documented that a significant percentage of patients suffering this injury never fully recover.[5–8] Between 19% and 72% of people who suffer an ankle

Disclosure: None.
Seal Beach Podiatry Group Inc, 550 Pacific Coast Highway, Suite 209, Seal Beach, CA 90174, USA
* Corresponding author.
E-mail address: drichiejr@aol.com

Clin Podiatr Med Surg 32 (2015) 195–215
http://dx.doi.org/10.1016/j.cpm.2014.11.003
0891-8422/15/$ – see front matter © 2015 Elsevier Inc. All rights reserved.

podiatric.theclinics.com

sprain suffer another sprain in the future.[9,10] Up to 70% of people suffering an ankle sprain develop long-term residual symptoms and/or a syndrome known as CAI.[8,11]

Patients with CAI have several residual symptoms that include feelings of giving way and instability, as well as repeated ankle sprains, persistent weakness, pain during activity, and self-reported disability.[12] There are 2 primary components of CAI: mechanical and functional. Mechanical instability is the result of pathologic laxity, impaired arthrokinematics, and joint degenerative changes.[13] Functional instability may be due to altered neuromuscular control, strength deficits, and deficient postural control.[14] All these components of CAI are thought to be preventable through a proper functional rehabilitation program.[15]

One reason that athletes develop permanent sequelae from an ankle sprain is because they may have returned to sport before they have fully recovered and healed their injury. The decision to return to sport is often made outside of the realm of a treating physician, where many different individuals such as coaches and athletic trainers with varying levels of expertise may be called upon to release the athlete to play. In other cases, a physician may be the only person whom the athlete may consult to obtain medical clearance.

For the podiatric physician who is facing an anxious parent seeking release of their adolescent athlete to return to the playing field, the decision-making process can be daunting. Because premature return to sport after an ankle sprain has a high likelihood of reinjury or permanent disability, what criteria can be used to assure that the proper decision is made? Are there objective measures that have been tested for reliability? Should athletes be allowed to give input, and if so, what information can they provide that is valuable and valid? What performance tests can be used to predict successful return to sport while minimizing the risk of CAI?

With increased focus on this critical issue of return-to-play (RTP) decision making among many disciplines in the sports medicine community, there is now a substantial amount of information and credible evidence that can aid the podiatric physician treating the ankle sprain in the athlete. This article reviews the essential components of the decision-making process and proposes useful criteria for implementation in podiatric practice.

DEFINITION

RTP is the process of deciding when an injured or ill athlete may safely return to practice or competition.[16] According to the consensus statement from the American College of Sports Medicine, the team physician must coordinate all levels of evaluation and treatment of the injured athlete and must have an RTP process in place before releasing the athlete to sport.[16] The team physician or the specialty podiatric physician may have a role in all of these processes:

- Evaluating injured or ill athletes
- Treating injured or ill athletes
- Rehabilitating injured or ill athletes
- Returning an injured or ill athlete to play

Each of these processes is briefly summarized, specific to the ankle sprain, with emphasis on the final evaluation and decision to return the athlete to play.

EVALUATION AND TREATMENT

Podiatric physicians may encounter patients immediately after suffering an ankle sprain or, more likely, at a later date when recovery has not been achieved and specialty referral has been sought. Whether the injury is acute or chronic, the responsibility of the treating physician is to thoroughly evaluate the sprain and determine the extent of injury. The key components of the evaluation process are history, physical examination, and imaging studies. An expert panel assembled by the National Athletic Trainers Association published a position paper on guidelines for the evaluation and treatment of the ankle sprain in athletes.[17] For podiatric physician this resource is an excellent comprehensive review of current evidence-based recommendations for the evaluation and treatment of the ankle sprain.

REHABILITATION

A proper rehabilitation program that follows evidence-based protocols and is individualized for the patient is critical to the recovery from an ankle sprain.[15] The podiatric physician must rely on the expertise of a skilled rehabilitation team who have experience and a commitment to providing a structured, progressive rehabilitation program for all patients referred for treatment of the ankle sprain. This team usually involves a physical therapist, a certified athletic trainer, or both.

The functional rehabilitation program for recovery from ankle sprain has 4 aspects: joint range of motion, muscular strengthening, proprioception, and activity-specific training.[17] Controversy has arisen regarding the timing of implementation of the functional rehabilitation program. Previously, encouraging joint range of motion and muscular strengthening would have been indicated from day 1, as long as the ankle joint was deemed stable.[18–20] However, studies of patients with CAI have provided insight about what factors should be addressed in a rehabilitation program. Hubbard and colleagues[21] studied 30 subjects with chronic ankle sprain and compared side-to-side differences and also compared healthy controls to determine which measures would most accurately predict CAI. Measures of mechanical laxity had the strongest relationship to CAI compared with functional measures. When comparing ankles with CAI to healthy controls, mechanical laxity was the most prevalent finding, explaining 31% of the variance between the groups; this led the researchers to question the current established protocols for early functional rehabilitation and quick return to sports activity.[21]

A systematic review by Kerkhoffs and colleagues[22] assessed the effectiveness of methods of immobilization for acute lateral ankle ligament injuries and compared immobilization with functional treatment methods. When low-quality trials were removed, there was no significant difference in outcome between early functional activity compared with immobilization of acute ankle sprains. Hubbard and colleagues[21] conclude that further research is necessary to determine if there is a relationship between early RTP and the risk of long-term mechanical instability.

PROTECTING THE ANKLE DURING RECOVERY

When studying the basic science of ligament repair, one can appreciate the length of time required for adequate healing after an ankle sprain. After initial ligament tear, 3 phases of healing must take place: inflammatory, proliferative, and maturation.[23] The maturation phase begins around day 21 after injury, whereas debate exists about how long it takes for ankle ligament repair to attain adequate strength to provide a stable ankle joint.[24] For the most part, prevailing standard of care of ankle sprains ignores the scientific evidence for the time frame required for adequate ligament repair and the athlete is returned to sport well before appropriate tissue healing has occurred.[25] Recurrent instability and reinjury can occur where healing is incomplete. If patients return to activity before the ligaments have fully healed, the ligament may heal in an elongated state. This elongated ligament state could result in increased joint movement (mechanical laxity), which may lead to the development of CAI.[26]

A systematic review of published studies treating ankle sprains revealed that mechanical laxity is seen in most subjects up to 1 year after suffering an ankle sprain.[27] Another study by Hubbard and Cordova[28] assessed the natural recovery of ankle ligament laxity after an acute lateral ankle sprain with an instrumented ankle arthrometer. The investigators quantified the anterior-posterior load displacement and inversion-eversion rotational laxity characteristics of the ankle-subtalar joint complex within 3 days after injury and again 8 weeks after injury. The results indicate that ankle laxity did not significantly decrease during 8 weeks, which suggests that the lateral ligaments of the ankle need to be protected for longer than 8 weeks if mechanical stability is to be restored after an acute lateral ankle sprain.

The requirements for protecting the ligaments of the ankle after a sprain remain a debated topic. Although prophylactic bracing when returning to sport has gained significant validity with recent studies, the type of brace or immobilizing device that best treats the acute sprain has not been agreed on.[22] A level 1 study has added more fuel to the controversy about immobilization after an ankle sprain.[29] This multicenter randomized trial studied 584 participants with severe ankle sprain who were treated with 3 different types of mechanical support. Patients who received the below-knee cast for 10 days had a more rapid recovery than those given the tubular compression bandage, an air stirrup brace, or a walking boot. The researchers concluded that, contrary to popular clinical opinion, a period of immobilization was the most effective strategy for promoting rapid recovery, which was achieved best by the application of a below-knee cast, an intervention that has previously been discouraged in favor of air stirrup braces.[25]

RESTORING NEUROMUSCULAR CONTROL

Ankle sprains cause direct damage not only to ligaments but also to the mechanoreceptors within the ligaments, joint capsule, and retinacula around the ankle joint, which provide afferent information to the central nervous system about joint movement and position.[30] This information is critical to the ability of a person to maintain postural control and balance during standing and running activities. Deficits in postural control are commonly observed after an acute ankle sprain.[31,32] Loss of proprioception is only one mechanism of loss of postural control after an ankle sprain. Delayed nerve conduction, strength deficits, and restricted joint range of motion have been measured after an ankle sprain and are part of the feed-forward or efferent side of neuromuscular control of the ankle.[33–37] An effective rehabilitation program should address all components of neuromuscular control, and deficits must be detected before an athlete is deemed ready to RTP.

Restoring neuromuscular control may incorporate a wide range of exercises and programs. The core of the rehabilitation program involves balance training on some type of wobble board or challenging device.[38,39] For example, a study by Wester and colleagues[40] showed that wobble-board training for 12 weeks starting 1 week after an acute ankle sprain would reduce the chance of reinjury by 50%. Another study by Holme and colleagues[41] showed that subjects who received balance training had a 3% reinjury rate compared with a 16% reinjury rate in the control group.

STRENGTH DEFICITS

Muscular strength is not only an important component of neuromuscular control but also essential for proper movement patterns when returning to sport. Strengthening and flexibility exercises are essential parts of the rehabilitation program treating the ankle sprain, but which muscle groups and which type of exercise to implement remain debated.[35] Although peroneal muscle weakness has been a popular focus of both causing and resulting from an acute ankle sprain, studies have questioned whether this is actually true.[42–44] Several studies have found that patients with functional ankle instability actually have loss of inversion rather than eversion strength.[45,46] Hubbard and colleagues[21] showed that patients with CAI have weakness of ankle plantar flexors. Rehabilitation programs now emphasize strengthening all muscle groups using both eccentric and concentric exercise.[47,48]

RETURN TO PLAY

Once evaluation, treatment, and rehabilitation of the injury has been completed, the treating physician ultimately has to make a decision whether the athlete is ready to return to sport. According to the position statement from the American College of Sports Medicine, the physician should confirm the following criteria when making an RTP decision:

- The status of anatomic and functional healing
- The status of recovery from acute illness and associated sequelae
- The status of chronic injury or illness
- That the athlete poses no undue risk to the safety of other participants
- Restoration of sport-specific skills
- Psychosocial readiness
- Ability to perform safely with equipment modification, bracing, and orthoses
- Compliance with applicable federal, state, local, school, and governing body regulations

Confirming all these factors can be challenging and time consuming for the treating physician. Receiving input from other members of the rehabilitation team is critical, as many of these factors cannot be monitored or measured in the physician clinic or practice setting. The podiatric physician may be part of a sports medicine team who provides input to the Team Physician who makes the ultimate RTP decision. Or, more often, the podiatric physician may be the sole decision maker particularly when treating a recreational athlete who is not part of organized sport.

The following section has been developed specifically for the podiatric physician who may be treating both high-level and casual recreational athletes. In either case, a decision to return to sport or activity is important and puts considerable responsibility on the podiatric physician.

SELF-REPORTED VARIABLES

Although most podiatric physicians would consider pain, swelling, and joint range of motion to be accurate indicators of recovery from an ankle sprain, studies have shown that none of these factors are reliable.[49] This result raises the question whether the patient rather than the clinician is in the best position to assess the status of recovery from an ankle sprain.[50] Outcomes research puts heavy emphasis on patient perception of function and quality of life relative to a disease or injury.[51] Self-reported outcomes instruments have been developed to help researchers and clinicians evaluate the effects of a pathologic condition or injury on physical function. These instruments can also be used to measure the effects of treatment of such a disease or injury. There are many instruments that have relevance to diseases or injuries to the lower extremity. In monitoring recovery from an ankle sprain, several instruments are relevant, including the

Foot and Ankle Disability Index,[52] Foot and Ankle Ability Measure (FAAM),[53] Lower Extremity Function Score,[54] and the Sports Ankle Rating System.[55]

These instruments are evaluative, as they are designed to measure an individual's change in health status over time.[56,57] The instruments have a scoring scale that can be used to quantify functional disability after an ankle sprain. The data generated can be useful for research but may be cumbersome for practical application in clinical practice. Several of these instruments have subsections that pose questions regarding ankle function during sport, which could not be used for RTP decision making since the athlete has not yet been cleared to play. Conversely, these instruments can provide useful guidelines for the clinician regarding key questions that must be asked of patients who are being evaluated for RTP after an ankle sprain. A review of the FAAM Activities of Daily Living Subscale reveals a comprehensive list of questions that can provide valid self-reported deficits associated with functional instability of the ankle (**Fig. 1**).[58]

A

Activities of Daily Living subscale

Please answer **every question** with **one response** that most closely describes to your condition within the past week.

If the activity in question is limited by something other than your foot or ankle mark **not applicable (N/A).**

	No difficulty	Slight difficulty	Moderate difficulty	Extreme difficulty	Unable to do	N/A
Standing	☐	☐	☐	☐	☐	☐
Walking on even ground	☐	☐	☐	☐	☐	☐
Walking on even ground without shoes	☐	☐	☐	☐	☐	☐
Walking up hills	☐	☐	☐	☐	☐	☐
Walking down hills	☐	☐	☐	☐	☐	☐
Going up stairs	☐	☐	☐	☐	☐	☐
Going down stairs	☐	☐	☐	☐	☐	☐
Walking on uneven ground	☐	☐	☐	☐	☐	☐
Stepping up and down curbs	☐	☐	☐	☐	☐	☐
Squatting	☐	☐	☐	☐	☐	☐
Coming up on your toes	☐	☐	☐	☐	☐	☐
Walking initially	☐	☐	☐	☐	☐	☐
Walking 5 minutes or less						
Walking approximately 10 minutes	☐	☐	☐	☐	☐	☐
Walking 15 minutes or greater	☐	☐	☐	☐	☐	☐

Fig. 1. (*A, B*) Foot and ankle ability measure—activities of daily living subscale.

B

Because of your foot and ankle how much difficulty do you have with:

	No difficulty at all	Slight difficulty	Moderate difficulty	Extreme difficulty	Unable to do	N/A
Home Responsibilities	☐	☐	☐	☐	☐	☐
Activities of daily living	☐	☐	☐	☐	☐	☐
Personal care	☐	☐	☐	☐	☐	☐
Light to moderate work (standing, walking)	☐	☐	☐	☐	☐	☐
Heavy work (push/pulling, climbing, carrying)	☐	☐	☐	☐	☐	☐
Recreational activities	☐	☐	☐	☐	☐	☐

How would you rate your current level of function during your usual activities of daily living from 0 to 100 with 100 being your level of function prior to your foot or ankle problem and 0 being the inability to perform any of your usual daily activities?

☐☐☐.0 %

Fig. 1. (*continued*).

The most useful ankle function evaluation protocol for application in podiatric practice is found in the Sports Ankle Rating System.[55] The authors have used parts of this system in their own practice for more than 10 years to make RTP decisions in athletes after an ankle sprain. The questionnaires should be administered to the patient in written form, and the patient should be given the opportunity to complete each section before the interview and examination are conducted by the physician. This method allows the patient time to reflect on each answer and provide a response that is not influenced by the health care providers or other interested parties.

The Sports Ankle Rating System starts with a patient-based questionnaire that evaluates the impact that an ankle injury has on the quality of life of the patient. Five questions are posed for 5 subscales. Of these, the questionnaires evaluating symptoms, activities of daily living, and lifestyle have proved to be the most valid and useful in podiatric practice (**Figs. 2–4**).

The second section of the Sports Ankle Rating System is a Clinical Rating Score, which is provided by both patient- and clinician-administered sections. The patient-based section consists of visual analog scales for pain, swelling, stiffness, giving-way, and function (**Fig. 5**). These questionnaires are useful for monitoring recovery and can be administered to the patient for completion at each office visit.

All valid patient self-assessment instruments contain a single global question about overall ankle joint function. In the FAAM, the question states "How would you rate your current level of function during your usual activities of daily living from 0 to 100, with 100 being your level of function prior to your foot or ankle problem and 0 being the inability to perform any of your usual daily activities?" The Sports Ankle Rating System uses the Single Assessment Numeric Evaluation whereby patients are asked to answer the following single written question: "On a scale of 0 to 100, how would you rate your ankle's function with 100 being normal?" A single question such as those

SPORTS ANKLE RATING SYSTEM
– QUALITY OF LIFE MEASURE

SCALE 1: **SYMPTOMS**

Instructions: Please circle the answer that best describes your ankle
symptoms **during the last week**

1. **How often was your ankle painful?**
2. **How often did you experience ankle swelling?**
3. **How often did your ankle feel stiff?**
4. **How often did your ankle feel weak?**
5. **How often did your ankle give way?**

Rate these 0 to 4 (4 being never or none)

0   1   2   3   4

Fig. 2. Sports ankle rating system—questionnaire for symptoms.

proposed should be included on the written questionnaire that is completed by the patient before the examination takes place.

FUNCTIONAL PERFORMANCE TESTING

When an athlete is deemed ready to return to play and when treatment has been determined to have been completed, several performance tests must be successfully completed. Many performance tests have been developed to identify patients with functional instability of the ankle, such as single hop for distance, shuttle run, side

SPORTS ANKLE RATING SYSTEM
QUALITY OF LIFE MEASURE
SCALE 1: ACTIVITIES OF DAILY LIVING

Instructions: Please circle the answer that **best** describes describes the
impact that your ankle had on your daily activities **during the last week**

1. How painful was your ankle during your daily activities?

2. How much difficulty did your ankle give you when you took care of yourself physically (for example, dressing or taking a shower?

3. How much difficulty did your ankle give you when you performed household chores?

4. How much did your ankle slow you down when you performed your daily activities?

5. How much did your ankle effect your ability to participate in your typical social activities?

Rate these 0 to 4 (4 being never or none)

0   1   2   3   4

Fig. 3. Sports ankle rating system—questionnaire for activities of daily living.

SPORTS ANKLE RATING SYSTEM QUALITY OF LIFE MEASURE
SCALE 1: **LIFESTYLE**

Instructions: Please circle the answer that best describes the impact that your ankle had on your lifestyle **during the last week.**

1. How much did your ankle effect your enjoyment of life?

2. How much confidence have you had in your ankle?

3. How often did your think about your ankle? (examples: my ankle hurts, my ankle won't let me...)

4. How much did your injured ankle limit your ability to do the things you wanted to do?

5. How much did lifestyle changes caused by your ankle (for example, not being able to do something you wanted to) effect your ability to enjoy spending time with other people?

Rate these 0 to 4 (4 being never or none)

0	1	2	3	4

Fig. 4. Sports ankle rating system—questionnaire for lifestyle.

SPORTS ANKLE RATING SYSTEM – CLINICAL RATING SCORE
SUBJECTIVE VISUAL ANALOG SCALES (Compiled by the Patient)

Instructions: Each line below represents a range of function in the item listed to its left (Pain, Swelling, Stiffness, Giving Way, and Function). The left end of each line indicates severe difficulty in the listed item and the right end of each line indicates perfect function in that item. Please draw a vertical line across the point on each line that represents the level of difficulty you have experienced with your ankle in each item during the past week. You may mark anywhere along each line.

EXAMPLE constant symptoms	no symptoms

PAIN   severe pain   no pain

SWELLING   severe swelling   no swelling

STIFFNESS   very stiff   no stiffness

GIVING WAY   gives way often   no giving way

FUNCTION   walking on level   totally normal
                        surface is difficult   ankle function

Fig. 5. Sports ankle rating system—clinical rating score: visual analog scales for pain, swelling, stiffness, giving-way, and function.

hop, and up-and-down hop.[59] Performance tests have not been specifically evaluated for appropriateness in making an RTP decision. The general recommendation is that when using functional testing and making an RTP decision, clinicians must compare the injured ankle with the uninvolved limb and determine that the injured ankle has achieved at least an 80% performance level.[11]

Measuring deficits in balance and postural control after an ankle sprain may be a more accurate way to monitor recovery.[60] The single-leg balance test (modified Romberg test) is the most simple and an easy test to administer in the clinic setting and has proved to be reliable in detecting balance deficits in athletes after an ankle sprain (**Fig. 6**).[61]

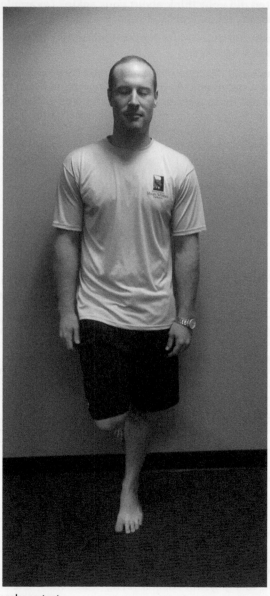

Fig. 6. Modified Romberg test.

However, researchers and clinicians have suggested that measures of dynamic balance are more reliable and predictive of recovery after an ankle sprain.[62] The Star Excursion Balance Tests are considered more accurate in assessing lower extremity function than static tests.[63–65] This test simultaneously measures strength, range of motion, proprioception, and neuromuscular control. The test is performed by having the athlete stand on one foot and then reach the contralateral foot in 8 predetermined directions. The test has been simplified to include only 3 reach directions: anteromedial, medial, and posteromedial (**Fig. 7**).[66] The podiatric physician can quickly implement this 3-reach test to measure dynamic balance when comparing the injured with the noninjured ankle.

Quantitative measurements are taken in all these tests, such as time to complete the task or distance achieved with hopping. Taking these measurements can be challenging in a podiatric physicians office, so the authors have selected those tests that have been most feasible to administer in this setting.

HOPPING

The lateral hop and the forward hop have both been tested and proved valid to identify residual disability after an ankle sprain.[11,67] Both tests are simple to perform in the

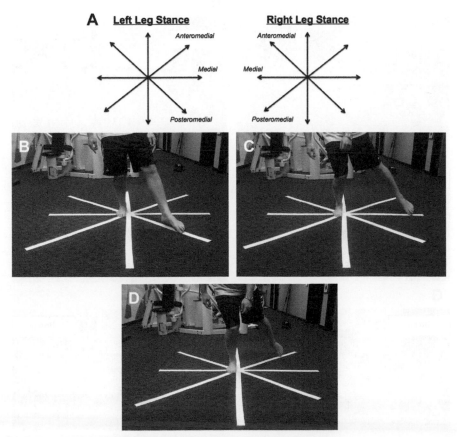

Fig. 7. (*A–D*) Modified star excursion balance test. The test has been simplified to include only 3 reach directions: anteromedial, medial, and posteromedial. (*Data from* Hertel J, Braham RA, Hale SA, et al. Simplifying the star excursion balance test: analyses of subjects with and without chronic ankle instability. J Orthop Sports Phys Ther 2006;36(3):131–7.)

clinic setting and do not require any specific measurement. For the lateral hop test, the patient is instructed to stand on the noninjured leg and then take 3 successive hops laterally or sideways down the hallway. From that end point, the patient then stands on the injured leg and is instructed to take 3 hops back in the reverse direction, hopping laterally. The test is successful if the patient returns to the original starting point with 3 hops on the injured leg (**Fig. 8**). For the forward hop test, the patient hops in an

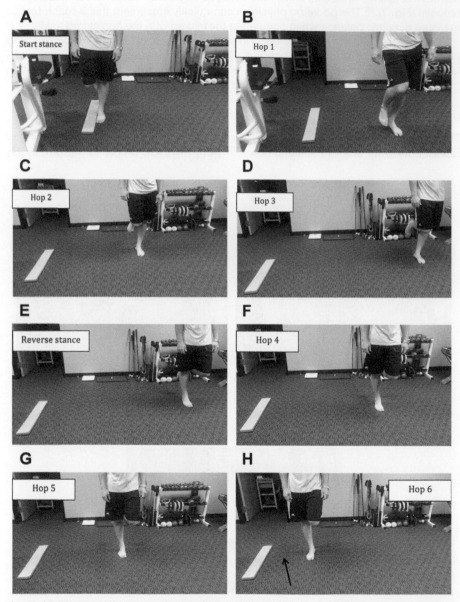

Fig. 8. (A–H) Lateral hop test. Patient first stands on uninjured leg and takes 3 successive lateral hops. From this end point, the patient then stands on the injured leg and is instructed to take 3 successive lateral hops back, with a goal of reaching the starting point. *Arrow* depicted in final figure shows failure of subject to reach the starting point on his injured leg.

anterior direction starting on the noninjured leg and then turns 180° and hops back 3 times on the injured leg (**Fig. 9**).

SINGLE LEG STANCE FOR TIME

The patient is instructed to fold both arms across the chest and stand on the noninjured foot for as long as possible, keeping the injured foot or ankle off the floor. A timer

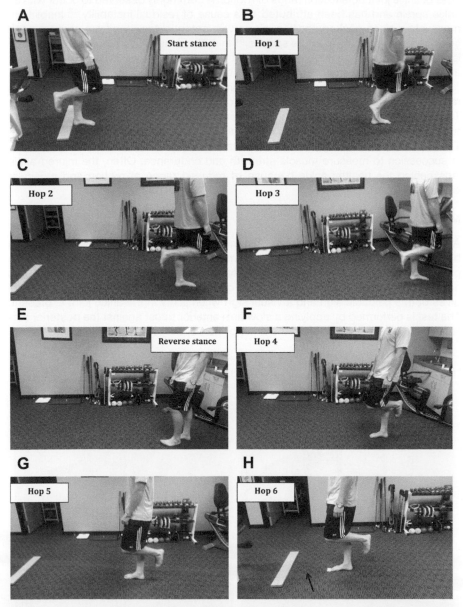

Fig. 9. (*A–H*) Forward hop test. Patient first stands on uninjured leg and takes 3 successive forward hops. From this end point, the patient turns 180° and takes 3 successive forward hops back on their injured leg, with a goal of reaching the starting point. *Arrow* depicted in final figure shows failure of subject to reach the starting point on his injured leg.

is used to record how long the task is held until balance is lost and the opposite foot touches the floor. Often, the patient is required to close the eyes to achieve an end point to the task with loss of balance. Comparison is then made to the contralateral, injured extremity (see **Fig. 6**).

HEEL ROCKERS

Loss of ankle joint dorsiflexion range of motion is commonly observed to occur with an ankle sprain and has been attributed to a cause of residual instability.[13] Inability to move into a close-packed position, along with potential toe drag from equinus positioning, can predispose to future sprains.[68] Inability of the talus to move into dorsiflexion after a sprain is thought to be the result of impaired anterior positioning of the talus, an anterior positional fault of the fibula, or both.[69,70]

The heel rocker test can provide a dynamic assessment of ankle joint dorsiflexion range of motion, as well as a measurement of lower leg dorsiflexion muscular strength. This test provides an instant side-to-side comparison of range of motion as the athlete rocks backward on the heels while raising the forefoot as far off the floor as possible. The patient should lean against a wall for stability and perform at least 10 heel rockers in succession to measure muscle strength and endurance. Often, the injured ankle lags behind the healthy ankle because of reduced range of motion and muscular strength (**Fig. 10**).

MANUAL TESTS FOR STABILITY

Anterior drawer and talar tilt are not only measured with radiographic stress imaging but can also be assessed via manual examination.[71] Laxity in the ankle joint can be palpated by a skilled examiner, particularly after the acute pain and swelling of the ankle joint have subsided.[72] The anterior drawer test is the easiest to perform and gives both a palpable sign and a visual sign when laxity in the ankle joint is present. The test is performed by applying a slow firm anterior thrust against the posterior surface of the heel while stabilizing the anterior part of the lower leg (**Fig. 11**).

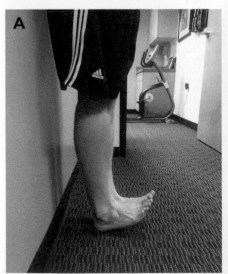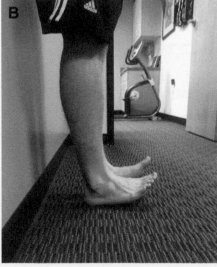

Fig. 10. (*A, B*) Heel rocker test. Often the injured ankle lags behind the healthy ankle because of reduced range of motion and muscular strength.

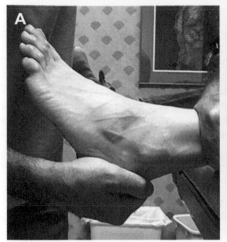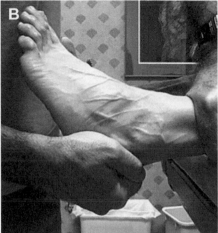

Fig. 11. (*A, B*) Anterior drawer test.

The manual talar tilt examination is traditionally performed with the patient supine to determine excessive inversion instability of the ankle joint. However, the authors have found that prone positioning can better evaluate side-to-side differences in combined ankle and rearfoot inversion. The calcaneal-fibular ligament is the primary soft-tissue restraint to both ankle and subtalar joint inversion, so the combined movement of these joints is best appreciated from a posterior view of the calcaneus (**Fig. 12**).

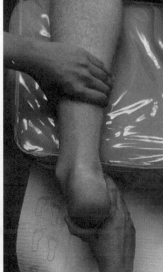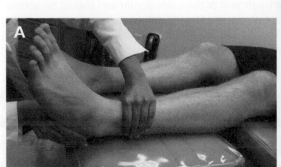

Fig. 12. (*A, B*) Clinical talar tilt test.

RESTORATION OF SPORT-SPECIFIC SKILLS

The final phase of rehabilitation of the ankle sprain involves activity-specific training. For the football player, this may mean running and cutting drills. For the volleyball player, this would include plyometric training with jumping maneuvers.[15] Implementing this phase of the training program relies on specialized physical therapists or athletic trainers with facilities and equipment that can simulate the sporting environment. Completion of this phase of training is done outside the realm of the treating physician, but assessment of mastery of sport-specific skills requires communication from the rehabilitation team so that the physician can make an RTP decision.[16]

BRACING AND ORTHOSES

The position paper from the American College of Sports Medicine cites the use of orthotics and braces as a primary consideration in the RTP decision.[16] The treating physician evaluates the need and prescribes orthoses and braces at any time during or after treatment of the ankle sprain.

FOOT ORTHOSES

Foot orthoses have shown a significant positive treatment effect for the athlete who has suffered an acute ankle sprain.[73] Several studies have demonstrated how foot orthoses can improve postural sway.[74,75] Other studies have specifically studied subjects after an acute ankle sprain and have shown that foot orthoses significantly reduced pain and improved postural control.[76,77] The mechanisms by which foot orthoses may achieve these treatment effects seem to be due to improved sensory feedback from the plantar surface of the foot, as well as improved positioning of the rearfoot for optimal muscular function.[73,78]

The studies of foot orthoses and treatment of ankle sprains have revealed positive effects for both custom-molded as well as prefabricated devices. In addition, several different designs of orthoses have been tested including semirigid and soft foam devices. Podiatric physicians are well trained to evaluate the foot type and biomechanical needs of the patient to prescribe and dispense foot orthoses to improve stability and recovery from an ankle sprain. At present, authorities from other disciplines are endorsing the use of foot orthoses as an important part of the treatment plan for rehabilitating the ankle sprain.[15,79]

ANKLE BRACES

Ankle braces are mandatory in the treatment of the ankle sprain and should be considered mandatory for use after the athlete returns to play. Although this recommendation might have been controversial 20 years ago, a significant body of research has been published that verifies the efficacy of prophylactic ankle bracing of the athlete when returning to sport after a sprain.

Ankle braces of different designs have been repeatedly shown to prevent the incidence of sprains in athletes in a variety of sports.[80–86] Taping is less effective than bracing in preventing ankle sprains.[81,87] For the current discussion, focus is on studies of athletes returning to sport after an ankle sprain. For these individuals, the scientific evidence is convincing that bracing has a protective effect in preventing a subsequent ankle sprain.[80,83,87,88] A systematic review demonstrated that athletes who had suffered a previous ankle sprain had 70% fewer ankle injuries when taped or braced compared with those who did not wear prophylactic support.[88]

In previous discussion the authors have shown the length of time required for liga-ments to heal adequately after rupture. From several studies, it can be concluded that after complete rupture, ankle ligaments have not achieved full strength until at least 6 months after injury.[6,8,23,27,28] Therefore, all athletes who have suffered significant lig-ament injury of the ankle should wear prophylactic ankle braces when returning to sport for a minimum of 6 months.

SUMMARY

Allowing the athlete to return to sport after injury involves a multifaceted decision-making process. For the ankle sprain, a large body of scientific evidence is now avail-able to provide a methodology for the podiatric physician in making an RTP decision. The patient must be provided self-assessment tools that have been tested for validity and reliability in detecting residual disability from the ankle sprain. Certain functional performance tests must also be administered to evaluate recovery and restoration of dynamic stability of the ankle joint. Finally, the podiatric physician should consider the benefits of implementing foot orthotic therapy and prophylactic ankle bracing to prevent reinjury in the athlete after returning to sport.

REFERENCES

1. Ferran NA, Maffulli N. Epidemiology of sprains of the lateral ankle ligament com-plex. Foot Ankle Clin 2006;11(3):659–62.
2. Kannus P, Renstrom P. Current concepts review: treatment for acute tears of the lateral ligaments of the ankle. J Bone Joint Surg Am 1991;73:305–12.
3. Birrer RB, Fani-Salek MH, Totten VY, et al. Managing ankle injuries in the emer-gency department. J Emerg Med 1999;17:651–60.
4. Rzonca EC, Lue BY. TEMPER: an acronym for ankle sprain rehabilitation. Clin Po-diatr Med Surg 1988;5:661–75.
5. Itay S, Ganel A. Clinical and functional status following lateral ankle sprains: follow-up of 90 young adults treated conservatively. Orthop Rev 1982;11:73–6.
6. Brand RL, Black HM, Cox JS. The natural history of inadequately treated ankle sprain. Am J Sports Med 1977;5:248–9.
7. Staples OS. Ruptures of the fibular collateral ligaments of the ankle: result study of immediate surgical treatment. J Bone Joint Surg Am 1975;57:101–7.
8. Verhagen RA, de Keizer G, van Dijk CN. Long-term follow-up of inversion trauma of the ankle. Arch Orthop Trauma Surg 1995;114:92–6.
9. Yeung MS, Chan KM, So CH, et al. An epidemiological survey on ankle sprain. Br J Sports Med 1994;28:112–6.
10. Braun BL. Effects of an ankle sprain in a generic clinical population 6 to 18 months after medical evaluation. Arch Fam Med 1999;8:143–8.
11. Gerber JP, Williams GN, Scoville CR, et al. Persistent disability associated with ankle sprains. Foot Ankle Int 1998;19:653–60.
12. Delahunt E, Coughlan GF, Caulfield B, et al. Inclusion criteria when investigating in-sufficiencies in chronic ankle instability. Med Sci Sports Exerc 2010;42(11):2106–21.
13. Delahunt E, Monaghan K, Caulfield B. Altered neuromuscular control and ankle joint kinematics during walking in subjects with functional instability of the ankle joint. Am J Sports Med 2006;34(12):1970–6.
14. Richie DH. Functional instability of the ankle and the role of neuromuscular con-trol: a comprehensive review. J Foot Ankle Surg 2001;40:240–51.
15. Mattacola CG, Dwyer MK. Rehabilitation of the ankle after acute sprain or chronic instability. J Athl Train 2002;37(4):413–42.

16. Herring S, Bergfeld J, Boyd J, et al. The team physician and return-to-play issues: a consensus statement. Med Sci Sports Exerc 2002;34(7):1212–4.

17. Kaminski TW, Hertel J, Amendola N, et al. National Athletic Trainers' Association position statement: conservative management and prevention of ankle sprains in athletes. J Athl Train 2013;48(4):528–45.

18. Andrews JR, Harrelson GL, Wilk KE. Physical rehabilitation of the injured athlete. 2nd edition. Philadelphia: WB Saunders; 1998.

19. Dettori JR, Pearson BD, Basmania CJ, et al. Early ankle mobilization, part I: the immediate effect on acute, lateral ankle sprains (a randomized clinical trial). Mil Med 1994;159:15–20.

20. Karlsson J, Lundin O, Lind K, et al. Early mobilization versus immobilization after ankle ligament stabilization. Scand J Med Sci Sports 1999;9:299–303.

21. Hubbard TJ, Kramer LC, Denegar CR, et al. Contributing factors to chronic ankle instability. Foot Ankle Int 2007;28:343–54.

22. Kerkhoffs GM, Rowe BH, Assendelft WJ, et al. Immobilisation and functional treatment for acute lateral ankle ligament injuries in adults. Cochrane Database Syst Rev 2002;(3):CD003762.

23. Andriacchi T, Sabiston P, DeHaven K, et al. Ligament: injury and repair. In: Woo SL, Buckwalter JA, editors. Injury and repair of the musculoskeletal soft tissues. Park Ridge (IL): American Academy of Orthopaedic Surgeons; 1987. p. 103–28.

24. Kannus P, Parkkary J, Jarvinen TA, et al. Basic science and clinical studies coincide: active treatment approach is needed after sports injury. Scand J Med Sci Sports 2003;13:150–4.

25. Beynnon BD, Renström PA, Haugh L, et al. A prospective, randomized clinical investigation of the treatment of first-time ankle sprains. Am J Sports Med 2006;34:1401–12.

26. Denegar CR, Miller SJ III. Can chronic ankle instability be prevented? Rethinking management of lateral ankle sprains. J Athl Train 2002;37(4):430–5.

27. Hubbard TJ, Hicks-Little CA. Ankle ligament healing after an acute ankle sprain. J Athl Train 2008;43(5):523–9.

28. Hubbard TJ, Cordova ML. Mechanical instability after an acute lateral ankle sprain. Arch Phys Med Rehabil 2009;90:1142–6.

29. Lamb SE, Marsh JL, Hutton JL, et al. Mechanical supports for acute, severe ankle sprain: a pragmatic, multicentre, randomised controlled trial. Lancet 2009;373: 575–81.

30. Freeman MA, Wyke BD. Articular reflexes at the ankle joint: an electromyographic study of normal and abnormal influences of ankle-joint mechanoreceptors upon reflex activity in the leg muscles. Br J Surg 1967;54:990–1001.

31. Garn SN, Newton RA. Kinesthetic awareness in subjects with multiple ankle sprains. Phys Ther 1988;68:1667–71.

32. Tropp H, Odenrick P. Postural control in single-limb stance. J Orthop Res 1988;6: 833–9.

33. Nitz AJ, Dobner JJ, Kersey D. Nerve injury and grades II and III ankle sprains. Am J Sports Med 1985;13:177–82.

34. Kleinrensink GJ, Stoeckart R, Meulstee J, et al. Lowered motor conduction velocity of the peroneal nerve after inversion trauma. Med Sci Sports Exerc 1994;26:877–83.

35. Lentell GL, Katzmann LL, Walters MR. The relationship between muscle function and ankle instability. J Orthop Sports Phys Ther 1990;11:605–11.

36. Pinstaar A, Brynhildsen J, Tropp H. Postural corrections after standardized perturbations of single leg stance: effect of training and orthotic devices in patients with ankle instability. Br J Sports Med 1996;30:151–5.

37. Isakov E, Mizrahi J. Is balance impaired by recurrent sprained ankle? Br J Sports Med 1997;31:65–7.
38. Gauffin H, Tropp H, Odendrick P. Effect of ankle disk training on postural control in patients with functional ankle instability of the ankle joint. Int J Sports Med 1988;9:141–4.
39. Hoffman M, Payne VG. The effects of proprioceptive ankle disk training on healthy subjects. J Orthop Sports Phys Ther 1995;21:90–3.
40. Wester JU, Jespersen SM, Nielsen KD, et al. Wobble board training after partial sprains of the lateral ligaments of the ankle: a prospective randomized study. J Orthop Sports Phys Ther 1996;23:332–6.
41. Holme E, Magnusson SP, Becher K, et al. The effect of supervised rehabilitation on strength, postural sway, position sense and re-injury risk after acute ankle ligament sprain. Scand J Med Sci Sports 1999;9(2):104–9.
42. Tropp H. Pronator muscle weakness in functional instability of the ankle joint. Int J Sports Med 1986;7:291–4.
43. Kaminski TW, Perrin DH, Gansneder BM. Eversion strength analysis of uninjured and functionally unstable ankles. J Athl Train 1999;34:239–45.
44. Bernier JN, Perrin DH, Rijke AM. Effect of unilateral functional instability of the ankle on postural sway and inversion and eversion strength. J Athl Train 1997; 32:226–32.
45. Munn J, Beard DJ, Refshauge KM, et al. Eccentric muscle strength in functional ankle instability. Med Sci Sports Exerc 2003;35:245–50.
46. Holmes A, Delahunt E. Treatment of common deficits associated with chronic ankle instability. Sports Med 2009;39(3):207–24.
47. Wilkerson GB, Pinerola JJ, Caturano RW. Invertor vs. evertor peak torque and power deficiencies associated with lateral ankle ligament injury. J Orthop Sports Phys Ther 1997;26:78–86.
48. Kaminski TW, Powers ME, Buckley BD, et al. The influence of strength and proprioception training on strength and postural stability in individuals with unilateral functional ankle instability [abstract]. J Athl Train 2001;36(Suppl):S-93.
49. Cross KM, Worrell TW, Leslie JE, et al. The relationship between self-reported and clinical measures and the number of days of return to sport following acute lateral ankle sprains. J Orthop Sports Phys Ther 2002;32:16–23.
50. Larmer PJ, NcNair PJ, Smythe L, et al. Ankle sprains: patient perceptions of function and performance of physical tasks. A mixed methods approach. Disabil Rehabil 2011;33:2299–304.
51. Landorf KB, Keenan AM. An evaluation of two foot-specific, health-related quality of life measuring instruments. Foot Ankle Int 2002;23(6):538–46.
52. Martin RL, Burdett RG, Irrgang JJ. Development of the foot and ankle disability index (FADI) [abstract]. J Orthop Sports Phys Ther 1999;29:32A–3A.
53. Martin RL, Irrgang JJ, Burdett RG, et al. Evidence of validity for the foot and ankle ability measure (FAAM). Foot Ankle Int 2005;26(11):968–83.
54. Alcock GK, Stratford PW. Validation of the lower extremity functional scale on athletic subjects with ankle sprains. Physiother Can 2002;54(4):233–40.
55. Williams GN, Molloy JM, DeBerardino TM, et al. Evaluation of the sports ankle rating system in young, athletic individuals with acute lateral ankle sprains. Foot Ankle Int 2003;24(3):274–82.
56. Kirshner B, Guyatt G. A methodological framework for assessing health indices. J Chronic Dis 1985;38(1):27–36.
57. Munn J, Beard DJ, Refshauge KM, et al. Do functional performance tests detect impairment in subjects with ankle instability? J Sport Rehabil 2002;11:40–50.

58. Carcia CR, Martin RL, Drouin JM. Validity of the foot and ankle ability measure in athletes with chronic ankle instability. J Athl Train 2008;43(2):179–83.
59. Buchanan AS, Docherty CL, Schrader J. Functional performance testing in participants with functional ankle instability and in a healthy control group. J Athl Train 2008;43(4):342–6.
60. Hertel J. Functional instability following lateral ankle sprain. Sports Med 2000;29: 361–71.
61. Kaikkonen A, Kannus P, Jarvinen M. A performance test protocol and scoring scale for the evaluation of ankle injuries. Am J Sports Med 1994;22(4):462–9.
62. Guskiewicz KM, Perrin DH. Research and clinical applications of assessing balance. J Sport Rehabil 1996;5:45–63.
63. Gray GW. Lower extremity functional profile. Adrian (MI): Wynn Marketing Inc; 1995.
64. Kinzey SJ, Armstrong CW. The reliability of the star-excursion test in assessing dynamic balance. J Orthop Sports Phys Ther 1998;27:356–60.
65. Hertel J, Miller SJ, Denegar CR. Intratester and intertester reliability during the star excursion balance tests. J Sport Rehabil 2000;9:104–16.
66. Hertel J, Braham RA, Hale SA, et al. Simplifying the star excursion balance test: analyses of subjects with and without chronic ankle instability. J Orthop Sports Phys Ther 2006;36(3):131–7.
67. Johnson MR, Stoneman PD. Comparison of a lateral hop test versus a forward hop test for functional evaluation of lateral ankle sprains. J Foot Ankle Surg 2007;46(3):162–74.
68. Drewes LK, McKeon PO, Kerrigan DC, et al. Dorsiflexion deficit during jogging with chronic ankle instability. J Sci Med Sport 2009;12(6):685–7.
69. Denegar CR, Hertel J, Fonseca J. The effect of lateral ankle sprain on dorsiflexion range of motion, posterior talar glide, and joint laxity. J Orthop Sports Phys Ther 2002;32(4):166–73.
70. Hubbard TJ, Hertel J. Anterior positional fault of the fibula after sub-acute lateral ankle sprains. Man Ther 2008;13(1):63–7.
71. Van Dijk CN, Mol BW, Lim LS, et al. Diagnosis of ligament rupture of the ankle joint: physical examination, arthrography, stress radiography and sonography compared in 160 patients after inversion trauma. Acta Orthop Scand 1996; 67(6):566–70.
72. Van Dijk CN, Lim LS, Bossuyt PM, et al. Physical examination is sufficient for the diagnosis of sprained ankles. J Bone Joint Surg Br 1996;78(6):958–62.
73. Richie DH. Effects of foot orthoses in the treatment of chronic ankle instability. J Am Podiatr Med Assoc 2007;97(1):19–30.
74. Ochsendorf DT, Mattacola CG, Arnold BL. Effect of orthotics on postural sway after fatigue of the plantar flexors and dorsiflexors. J Athl Train 2000;35:26–30.
75. Miller AK, Mattacola CG, Uhl TL, et al. Effect of orthotics on postural stability over a six week acclimation period [abstract]. J Athl Train 2001;36(Suppl):S-67.
76. Guskiewicz KM, Perrin DH. Effect of orthotics on postural sway following inversion ankle sprain. J Orthop Sports Phys Ther 1996;23:326–31.
77. Orteza LC, Vogelbach WD, Denegar CR. The effect of molded and unmolded orthotics on balance and pain while jogging following inversion ankle sprain. J Athl Train 1992;27:80–4.
78. Kavounoudias A, Roll R, Roll JP. The plantar sole is a 'dynamometric map' for human balance control. Neuroreport 1998;9:3247–52.
79. Hertel J, Denegar C, Buckley WE, et al. Effect of rear-foot orthotics on postural control in healthy subjects. J Sport Rehabil 2001;10:36–47.

80. Tropp H, Askling C, Gillquist J. Prevention of ankle sprains. Am J Sports Med 1985;13(4):259–62.
81. Rovere G, Clarke T, Yates C, et al. Retrospective comparison of taping and ankle stabilizers in preventing ankle injuries. Am J Sports Med 1988;16(3):228–33.
82. Mickel TJ, Bottoni CR, Tsuji G, et al. Prophylactic bracing versus taping for the prevention of ankle sprains in high school athletes: a prospective, randomized trial. Foot Ankle Surg 2006;45(6):360–5.
83. Surve I, Schwellnus MP, Noakes T, et al. A fivefold reduction in the incidence of recurrent ankle sprains in soccer players using Sport-Stirrup orthosis. Am J Sports Med 1994;22(5):601–6.
84. Sharpe SR, Knapik J, Jones B. Ankle braces effectively reduce recurrence of ankle sprains in female soccer players. J Athl Train 1997;32(1):21–4.
85. Sitler M, Ryan J, Wheeler B, et al. The efficacy of a semirigid ankle stabilizer to reduce acute ankle injuries in basketball: a randomized clinical study at West Point. Am J Sports Med 1994;22(4):454–61.
86. Stasinopoulos D. Comparison of three preventive methods in order to reduce the incidence of ankle inversion sprains among female volleyball players. Br J Sports Med 2004;38(2):182–5.
87. Olmsted LC, Vela LI, Denegar CR, et al. Prophylactic ankle taping and bracing: a numbers-needed-to-treat and cost-benefit analysis. J Athl Train 2004;39(1):95–100.
88. Dizon JM, Reyes JJ. A systematic review on the effectiveness of external ankle supports in the prevention of inversion ankle sprains among elite and recreational players. J Sci Med Sport 2010;13(3):309–17.

Dynamic Techniques for Clinical Assessment of the Athlete

Alex Kor, DPM, MS*

KEYWORDS

- Ankle and foot • Physical examination • Ankle syndesmosis • Lateral ankle sprain
- Achilles tendon • Range of motion • Return to play • Stress fracture

KEY POINTS

- As the emphasis on controlling health care costs intensifies, the sports medicine provider needs to be equipped to minimize unnecessary tests.
- Reproducible clinical diagnostic tools can reduce imaging costs for athletes with foot and ankle conditions.
- Physical examination techniques should allow the athlete's medical team a thorough evaluation before the season, after an injury occurs, and on considering return-to-play scenarios.

INTRODUCTION

For a sports medicine provider, proper evaluation of the athlete who is experiencing (or has had) foot and ankle pain is essential in determining management and treatment. Whether the athlete is being screened before the season, needs to return to play after an injury, or needs to be cleared to play (or practice) after surgery or an injury, the provider must have access to a systematic and reproducible process for such an evaluation. As health care costs continue to rise, sports medicine providers must be cognizant that unnecessary use of resources can be avoided.[1] Therefore, it is imperative that a thorough history be obtained from the athlete, trainer, family member, and so forth. Gomez and colleagues[2] estimated that 92% of all musculoskeletal conditions can be detected by history alone. After that history is completed, a sports-specific

The author has nothing to disclose. No funding was received in support of this work.
Department of Orthopaedic Surgery, The Johns Hopkins University, Baltimore, MD, USA
* c/o Elaine P. Henze, BJ, ELS, Medical Editor and Director, Editorial Services, Department of Orthopaedic Surgery, Johns Hopkins Bayview Medical Center, The Johns Hopkins University, 4940 Eastern Avenue, #A665, Baltimore, MD 21224-2780.
E-mail address: akor1@jhmi.edu

and joint-specific examination (correlated with the history) should secure the correct diagnosis in an even higher percentage of athletes.[3]

PHYSICAL EXAMINATION OF THE LOWER EXTREMITY

Because the cause of most foot and ankle conditions is local, a thorough physical examination will focus primarily on the ankle and foot. However, in recent years, there has been more of a global approach to diagnosing and managing these lower extremity injuries.[4] This shift in evaluating musculoskeletal conditions emphasizes the identification of proximal (seemingly unrelated) and/or distal regions that may or may not be causative. Developed in 2007 and known as the regional interdependence model (**Fig. 1**), it allows the sports medicine team to provide a comprehensive approach to assessment, management, and return-to-play criteria. After the primary foot and ankle condition is examined, regions proximal and distal are also examined. As sports medicine podiatrists and members of the sports medicine team, foot and ankle specialists can request input from other providers regarding these proximal areas (eg, lower back, hip, or knee) that may be contributing to the foot and ankle condition. For example, if an athlete presents with forefoot pain that is localized to the third interspace of the affected foot, the diagnosis may be a Morton neuroma. Using the regional interdependence model, the examination would not be localized to the foot and ankle. Knowing that the forefoot is subject to overuse and that most athletes function in a closed kinetic chain, examination of the knee, hip, lower back, and their soft-tissue attachments should be included. David Craig, ATC, former trainer of the National Basketball Association's Indiana Pacers, has found a high correlation between overuse conditions of the foot and ankle and sacroiliac joint dysfunction (David Craig, personal communication, August 31, 2014). Renaming this concept "regional interdependence," Craig and others, including Swartzlander[5] and Hesch,[6] have been examining and successfully treating proximal regions for more distal pain.

When used in concert with this comprehensive approach, functional movement assessment provides better analysis and prediction of deficits that may result in injury or reinjury than when it is used alone. Known as the Functional Movement Screen, it uses 7 clinical and reproducible tests that challenge the athlete[7] (tests are available at: http://www.befittherapy.com/pdf/functional-movement-screen.pdf). Using a scoring system (eg, 0–3 for a total score of 21), the athlete is tested on a deep squat, hurdle step, in-line lunge,

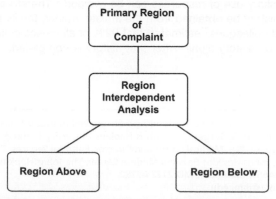

Fig. 1. The regional interdependence model. (*From* Cheatham S, Kreiswirth E. The regional interdependence model: a clinical examination concept. Int J Athl Ther Train 2014;19(3):9. Fig. 1; with permission.)

shoulder mobility, active straight leg raise, trunk stability push-up, and rotary stability. Regardless of the foot and ankle condition, some observers[8–10] have found that measuring the athlete's proprioception, mobility, and stability can assist the sports medicine team in allowing for better performance and less injury. Conversely, Warren and colleagues[11] recently concluded that functional movement screen, movement patterns, and asymmetry were poor predictors of musculoskeletal injuries in 167 Division I athletes. In that study, only the in-line lunge was associated with injury.

PHYSICAL EXAMINATION

Most lower extremity physical examinations are divided into 4 portions:

- Dermatologic
- Vascular
- Neurologic
- Musculoskeletal (see later discussion).

Nevertheless, inspection and palpation of the foot and ankle are the first parts of the physical examination that the health care provider will have with the athlete's foot or ankle condition. This gross examination will include a visual assessment of effusion, ecchymosis, edema, and skin integrity. After the initial cursory visual examination, the sports medicine podiatrist must properly assess the athlete's neurovascular status by palpating the pedal pulses and documenting the capillary refill of the digits of both feet. The examiner also needs to compare the affected and contralateral limbs in terms of the deep tendon reflexes, sensation, and presence or absence of a positive Tinel sign. In addition to the previously mentioned visual inspection of the skin, close attention to location and size of hyperkeratosis on both feet can provide valuable information for the astute clinician. In particular, the size and location of these plantar lesions strongly correlate with certain overuse injuries. A physical examination of the lower extremity is not complete without an analysis of gait.[12] Regardless of the sport, a walking and/or running gait analysis of the athlete can be useful in detecting a limb-length discrepancy, biomechanical errors, muscular imbalance, and so forth. Another overlooked opportunity to evaluate the athlete is a shoe gear assessment in which shoes are critiqued for sizing, wear patterns, toe break flexibility, torsional flexibility, and the rigidness of the shank.[12] Although efforts to make the evaluation of an athletic shoe more objective may not yet be successful, this evaluation should not be ignored.

MUSCULOSKELETAL EXAMINATION OF THE ANKLE

There is little doubt that the ankle is the most commonly injured body part in athletic populations.[13] Among this population, Stiell and colleagues[14] found that less than 15% actually have a fracture. Therefore, if the sports medicine provider can use the full complement of diagnostic clinical tests available, imaging costs may be substantially reduced and the athlete may be able to return to play sooner.

Injury to the distal tibiofibular (**Fig. 2**) ligament (or ankle syndesmosis) is underdiagnosed and underreported, but it can be quite disabling to the athlete.[15] This ligament provides inherent stability for the ankle mortise and consists of the interosseous ligament and the anterior and posterior inferior tibiofibular ligaments.[16] The typical mechanism that results in an injury to the ankle syndesmosis is a dorsiflexion and eversion force. Palpable tenderness and swelling are found at the level of the syndesmosis and just proximal to the syndesmosis. Usually, the range of motion is limited by guarding and the deformity. Whether the athlete is examined on the field (at the site of the event)

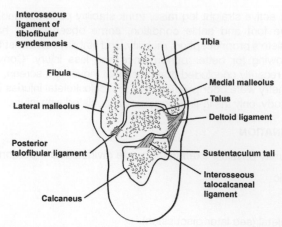

Fig. 2. Distal tibiofibular ligament (ankle syndesmosis). (*Courtesy of* The Johns Hopkins University, Baltimore, MD; with permission.)

or in a clinical setting, there are 4 clinical tests that can help in confirming this diagnosis[17,18]:

- External rotation (Kleiger) test
- Squeeze test
- Cotton test
- Fibular translation test.

The external rotation (or Kleiger) test (**Fig. 3**) is performed with the ankle joint in neutral position. The examiner places a hand to stabilize the proximal tibia and fibula and with the other hand exerts an eversion moment. Anterior ankle pain is suspicious for a syndesmotic injury. The squeeze test (**Fig. 4**) involves midcalf compression of the tibia and fibula. This proximal squeeze in the setting of an ankle syndesmotic injury results in pain of the ankle. Both of these tests will likely be negative with a lateral ankle sprain and positive with an ankle syndesmotic injury. These tests are not designed to necessarily reproduce pain. Rather, the Cotton test applies medial and lateral forces on the talus in a neutral positioned ankle. When compared with the asymptomatic limb, the Cotton test is deemed positive when this mediolateral motion is increased on the symptomatic side. Similarly, the fibular translation test applies an anterior-posterior force on the fibula in the hopes of finding an appreciable difference between the ankles. Various examiners have attempted to compare these tests.[19–21] Nussbaum and colleagues[21] found that the squeeze test was the only test applicable in a clinical setting and that a positive squeeze test was consistent with a poor prognosis for an earlier return to sport. In 2013, Sman and colleagues[18] agreed that the squeeze test had clinical relevance but concluded that there is no single test that should determine whether or not a syndesmotic ankle injury has occurred. In addition, they urged providers to be aware that these tests lack diagnostic sensitivity and specificity. Therefore, the provider needs to use these tests as an adjunct in conjunction with the history and subjective symptoms in determining an accurate diagnosis.

The more frequent lateral ankle sprain[17] usually involves 1 or more of the 3 lateral ankle ligaments:

- Anterior talofibular ligament (weakest)
- Calcaneofibular ligament
- Posterior talofibular ligament (strongest).

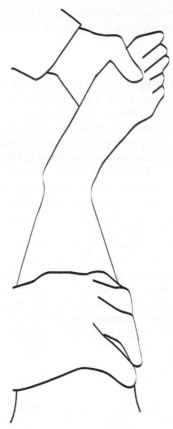

Fig. 3. The external rotation (or Kleiger) test. (*Courtesy of* The Johns Hopkins University, Baltimore, MD, USA; with permission.)

The typical mechanism, which includes an inversion motion of the foot and ankle, can occur when the athlete lands on another athlete's foot. Immediate pain, swelling, and difficulty in applying weight to the affected foot are the hallmarks of this injury. Often, these injuries occur when an immediate decision to return to play must be made.

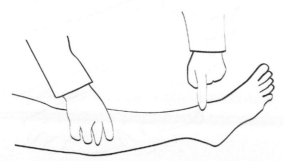

Fig. 4. The squeeze test. (*Courtesy of* The Johns Hopkins University, Baltimore, MD, USA; with permission.)

Therefore, the sports medicine provider should be knowledgeable about the 2 clinical tests that can assess the integrity of the lateral ankle ligaments:

- Anterior drawer test
- Talar tilt test

The anterior drawer test (**Fig. 5**) examines the degree of injury to the anterior talofibular ligament. The athlete is seated with the knee flexed at 90° and the ankle is plantarflexed by approximately 10° as the clinician applies an anterior force to the back of the heel with 1 hand while stabilizing the distal tibia with the other hand. The amount of anterior translocation of the talus on the remainder of the ankle joint and pain reproduced during the examination have been considered to be consistent with the degree of the injury (eg, grade I, II, or III).[22] Unfortunately, Croy and colleagues[23] concluded that the anterior drawer test has little clinical significance unless the examinations of the affected and contralateral limbs are compared and other physical measures are included. Typically, a 4-mm difference between the injured and uninjured ankle is considered clinically significant. The second test that is used when an athlete sustains a lateral ankle sprain is the talar tilt test (**Fig. 6**). Performed with the examiner's hands in the same position as the anterior drawer test, the hand holding the back of the heel inverts the affected foot. This test is designed to evaluate the integrity of the calcaneofibular ligament; however, many investigators[24–26] have found that the talar tilt is not as reliable as the anterior drawer test unless the results in the affected ankle are compared with those in the contralateral ankle. Previously, it was thought that for every 5° of inversion reproduced, the magnitude of the ankle sprain increased from primary to grade 2 and then grade 3.[24–26] Unfortunately, in recent years, this finding has not proven to be reliable.[22]

The longest and strongest tendon in the body is the Achilles tendon.[27] As with any soft-tissue structure, this tendon is prone to overuse and acute injury, which results in a complete or partial rupture of the substance of the tendon, usually 5 to 7 cm proximal to the insertion in the posterior portion of the calcaneus. The typical scenario when an athlete experiences an acute tear is the perception that he or she was "kicked in the back of the leg." In addition to the patient's inability to plantarflex the foot versus resistance, the Thompson test is highly reproducible (**Fig. 7**).[28,29] With the athlete prone on an examination table with both legs suspended off of the table, the calf of the affected

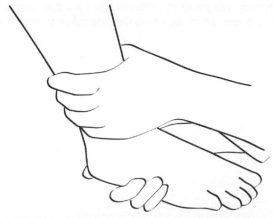

Fig. 5. The anterior drawer test. (*Courtesy of* The Johns Hopkins University, Baltimore, MD; with permission.)

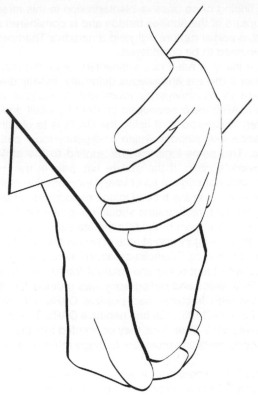

Fig. 6. The talar tilt test. (*Courtesy of* The Johns Hopkins University, Baltimore, MD; with permission.)

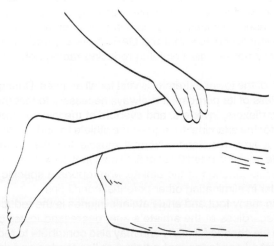

Fig. 7. The Thompson test. (*Courtesy of* The Johns Hopkins University, Baltimore, MD; with permission.)

leg is squeezed. A finding of no passive plantarflexion in this affected foot is highly consistent with a rupture of the Achilles tendon and is considered a positive Thompson test.[30] At times, a partial rupture will yield a negative Thompson test, and other diagnostic measures need to be considered.

Once a soft-tissue injury is ruled out, suspected, or confirmed, the clinician may also need to decipher if there is an osseous deformity. Initially developed to assess patients who present to an emergency room with a possible ankle fracture, the Ottawa ankle rules (OARs) were developed in 1992 by Stiell and colleagues[14] and modified a year later. The purpose of using the OARs is to obtain objective clinical findings that may accurately pinpoint which emergency room patients do or do not require radiographs. This same logic can be applied to the athlete in the training room or in the provider's clinic. If the athlete has pain in the malleolar zone and bone tenderness at posterior edge or tip of lateral (or malleolar) malleolus or is unable to bear weight after injury or at the time of injury, radiographs of the ankle should be ordered. Regarding the foot, radiographs should be ordered if the athlete has pain in the midfoot region and either pain of the fifth metatarsal base or navicular bone or is unable bear weight after the injury and at time of presentation.[31] In 2013, a study from the Tehran University of Medical Sciences assessed the accuracy of the OARs in athletes who presented with blunt ankle and midfoot fractures.[32] In that study, 2 clinicians examined 1156 athletes and radiography was ordered for all. They found that 100% of the athletes with fractures had positive OARs. Of the radiographs that were negative for a fracture (1165), 439 had negative OARs. The approximate net savings in radiographs was 33%. Therefore, they concluded that the use of the OARs is a reliable option for sports medicine providers to triage athletes with ankle and midfoot trauma.

The literature is not 100% unanimous in support of the OARs. In 2003, Glas and colleagues[33] compared the ability of surgical residents to use the OARs versus the Leiden ankle rules,[34] a system composed of 7 variables, versus physician judgment to correctly triage 690 subjects. They found that the sensitivity was 89% for the OARs, 80% for the Leiden ankle rules, and 82% for the residents' judgment. Specificity was found to be 26%, 59%, and 68%, respectively. In addition, missed fractures among the 3 groups numbered 8 for the OARs, 15 for the Leiden ankle rules, and 13 for the physicians. The conclusion reached in this study was that the clinical judgment of relatively inexperienced physicians-in-training compared favorably to established criteria in properly evaluating patients in a busy emergency room. Therefore, despite the well-established role that the OARs have enjoyed, this study suggests that these rules may not be that helpful in reducing radiography in lower extremity trauma.

Muscle strength of the lower extremity is vital for all athletes. During an athlete's examination, regardless of its purpose, it is always necessary to test the strength of the dorsiflexors, plantarflexors, inverters, and evertors of the lower extremity. A common method (**Fig. 8**) is for the examiner to request the athlete to perform the desired motion against gentle, but firm, resistance. Normal muscle function is rated 5 out of 5, whereas no muscle power is rated 0 out of 5. In conjunction with taking a good history, evaluating the muscle function of the athlete who reports a specific traumatic event can aid the provider in eliminating other potential conditions.

Another factor in many foot and ankle athletic injuries is the reduced range of motion measured. Regardless of the athlete's age, decreased lower extremity motion will likely increase the chance for injury and may also contribute to recurrent episodes of pain. It is common knowledge that a tight Achilles tendon and limited ankle joint range of motion are implicated as causative factors in many foot and ankle

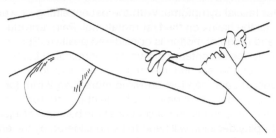

Fig. 8. Manual testing for muscle strength. (*Courtesy of* The Johns Hopkins University, Baltimore, MD; with permission.)

conditions, including lateral ankle sprains and forefoot pain.[35] Ankle joint measurement can be performed in a weight-bearing model (eg, controlled lunge) versus the more common non–weight-bearing method (knee extended vs knee flexed). However, the reliable and consistent measurement of ankle joint range of motion has been a source of confusion for an extended period. Wilken and colleagues[36] developed the Iowa ankle range of motion device (University of Iowa, Iowa City, IA, USA) (**Fig. 9**) that attempted to provide a standardized, reproducible apparatus for measuring ankle joint range of motion. Despite their acknowledgment that the study did not include ankle joints with known abnormality, the investigators concluded their apparatus provides a low-cost and effective option to objectively measure ankle joint range of motion.

As previously discussed, the OARs have been used for more than 20 years to minimize health care costs for ankle and midfoot trauma. Surprisingly, there are no other such well-established clinical criteria in guiding the clinician when an athlete presents with other sports medicine injuries, including those of the shoulder,[37] Lisfranc joint, and forefoot. Beyond paying close attention to the patient's history and performing a thorough physical examination that includes unreliable stress testing, the sports medicine provider needs to incorporate imaging much sooner in the evaluation of an athlete. Thus, future investigation is needed in an effort to develop reliable objective tests that primarily focus on the Lisfranc joint and forefoot.

Conversely, there are diagnostic tests that have been used to assess foot function and stability that have enjoyed varying degrees of acceptance. The windlass test,[12] more commonly implemented by physical therapists, is used to assess for the

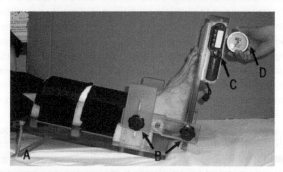

Fig. 9. The Iowa ankle range of motion device. (*A*) Knee flexion angle, (*B*) device axis of rotation, (*C*) angular displacement, and (*D*) known torque levels. (*From* Wilken J, Rao S, Estin M, et al. A new device for assessing ankle dorsiflexion motion: reliability and validity. J Orthop Sports Phys Ther 2011;41(4):275. Fig. 1; with permission.)

presence of plantar fascial symptoms. With the patient sitting or weight bearing, the examiner dorsiflexes the hallux on the first metatarsal. Pain reproduced in the plantar fascia before the end range of motion is considered positive. Sports medicine podiatrists more commonly use the anterior drawer test or modified Lachman test to assess the plantar capsule of the second metatarsophalangeal joint. A positive anterior drawer test or modified Lachman test showing more than 2 mm (or more than 50%) dorsal excursion is considered suggestive of a plantar plate rupture.[38]

Once an athlete has missed playing or practice time because of injury or subsequent surgery, a return-to-play decision will need to be considered by the entire sports medicine team. There is considerable debate about what process is best for determining this status for the athlete with an ankle injury[39,40] and clinicians are reluctant to use specific objective measurements as the sole factor in making this decision. However, clinicians do agree that the goals are to do no harm and to ensure that the athlete does not have pain, has no instability, and has near-symmetrical range of motion and strength.[41] For the lower extremity, there are well-known parameters that indicate when an athlete can be allowed to return to action after having anterior cruciate ligament reconstruction. Conversely, there are no such objective studies that can guide the sports medicine provider after a lateral ankle stabilization procedure is performed.

Stress fractures of the lower extremity are common in most impact-related sports; it is estimated that 10% of running injuries are stress fractures.[42] Once the diagnosis of a stress fracture is secured, there is no specific objective measurement that can assist the clinician in determining management of the injury. However, there is a general philosophy that should be adopted by all providers. Lower extremity stress fractures can be classified as high risk and low risk by studying biomechanics, natural history, and location. High-risk stress fractures include the sesamoids, fifth metatarsal base, navicular, medial malleolus, anterior tibia, and talar neck. Low risk stress fractures include the central 3 metatarsals, lateral malleolus, calcaneus, and femoral shaft. Kaeding and colleagues[42] concluded that the undertreatment of high-risk stress fractures can result in catastrophic outcomes with additional lost playing time. On the other hand, overtreatment of low-risk lower extremity stress fractures can produce an underconditioned athlete with unnecessary time away from his or her chosen sport. This delicate balance needs to be learned over time.

SUMMARY/DISCUSSION

This article reviewed clinical and diagnostic objective tests that allow the sports medicine provider to better assess the athlete with lower extremity conditions. Whether the athlete is examined on the field, in the locker room, or in the office, these tests have the potential to provide an early and accurate diagnosis, initiate a treatment and management regimen, and limit imaging costs. As Stiell and colleagues[14] discussed, less than 15% of ankle injuries are actually fractures. Therefore, to assist in lowering health care costs (ie, less imaging unless clearly justified), a sports medicine provider needs to be able to differentiate a fracture from a sprain or a ligament tear from a sprain. Unfortunately, there are some limitations to how much information can be garnered by the provider in assessing the athlete; only the squeeze test is known to be helpful in evaluating a high ankle sprain. When evaluating the athlete with a lateral ankle sprain, there is little agreement on the reliability of the anterior drawer test and the talar tilt test. Further investigation is needed to develop a better method to triage the lateral ankle sprain. Conversely, the Thompson test is an accepted way to assess the injured Achilles tendon. In addition, the OARs, used for more than 20 years, provide the sports medicine clinician with a useful tool in evaluating ankle and midfoot injuries. When treating forefoot athletic injuries, there are few objective examinations (excluding the modified Lachman test) that aid the sports medicine provider. In summary, as Gomez and colleagues[2] pointed out, most musculoskeletal injuries can be diagnosed by history alone. However, when the history alone is not sufficient, the provider with excellent clinical acumen will include the dynamic clinical assessment of the athlete in his or her armamentarium, recognizing the tests' limitations.

ACKNOWLEDGMENTS

This article would not have been possible without the assistance and encouragement offered by Elaine P. Henze, BJ, ELS, Jenni Weems, and Eileen Martin. In addition, I would like to thank Christine Caufield-Noll, Linda Gorman, Tillie Horak, and Rick Tracey for their contributions.

REFERENCES

1. Long AS, Scifers JR. Clinical prediction rules for diagnostic imaging after lower extremity trauma. Int J Athl Ther Train 2011;16:38–41.
2. Gomez JE, Landry GL, Bernhardt DT. Critical evaluation of the 2-minute orthopedic screening examination. Am J Dis Child 1993;147:1109–13.
3. Garrick JG. Preparticipation orthopedic screening evaluation. Clin J Sport Med 2004;14:123–6.
4. Cheatham S, Kreiswirth E. The regional interdependence model: a clinical examination concept. Int J Athl Ther Train 2014;19:8–14.
5. Swartzlander B. Outside the box: investigating a new model of assessing musculoskeletal disorder. ADVANCE 2008;19:62. Available at: http://physical-therapy.advanceweb.com/Features/Article-2/Revisiting-System-Independence.aspx.
6. Hesch J. Evaluation and treatment of the most common pattern of sacroiliac joint dysfunction. In: Vleeming A, Mooney V, Dorman T, et al, editors. Movement, stability, and low back pain—the essential role of the pelvis. New York: Churchill Livingstone; 1997. p. 535–45.
7. Teyhen DS, Shaffer SW, Lorenson CL, et al. The functional movement screen: a reliability study. J Orthop Sports Phys Ther 2012;42:530–40.
8. Chorba RS, Chorba DJ, Bouillon LE, et al. Use of a functional movement screening tool to determine injury risk in female collegiate athletes. N Am J Sports Phys Ther 2010;5:47–54.
9. Clover J, Wall J. Return-to-play criteria following sports injury. Clin Sports Med 2010;29:169–75.
10. Kiesel K, Plisky PJ, Voight ML. Can serious injury in professional football be predicted by a preseason functional movement screen? N Am J Sports Phys Ther 2007;2:147–58.
11. Warren M, Smith CA, Chimera NJ. Association of functional movement screen with injuries in division I athletes. J Sport Rehabil 2014. [Epub ahead of print].
12. Rao S, Riskowski JL, Hannan MT. Musculoskeletal conditions of the foot and ankle: assessments and treatment options. Best Pract Res Clin Rheumatol 2012;26:345–68.
13. Fernandez WG, Yard EE, Comstock RD. Epidemiology of lower extremity injuries among U.S. high school athletes. Acad Emerg Med 2007;14:641–5.
14. Stiell IG, Greenberg GH, McKnight RD, et al. A study to develop clinical decision rules for the use of radiography in acute ankle injuries. Ann Emerg Med 1992;21:384–90.

15. Gerber JP, Williams GN, Scoville CR, et al. Persistent disability associated with ankle sprains: a prospective examination of an athletic population. Foot Ankle Int 1998;19:653–60.
16. Mahadevan V. Ankle and foot. In: Strandring S, editor. Gray's anatomy: the anatomical basis of clinical practice. 40th edition. Philadelphia: Churchill Livingstone; 2008. p. 1429–62.
17. Hang B. Acute sports-related lower extremity injuries. Clin Pediatr Emerg Med 2013;14:304–17.
18. Sman AD, Hiller CE, Refshauge KM. Diagnostic accuracy of clinical tests for diagnosis of ankle syndesmosis injury: a systematic review. Br J Sports Med 2013;47:620–8.
19. Alonso A, Khoury L, Adams R. Clinical tests for ankle syndesmosis injury: reliability and prediction of return to function. J Orthop Sports Phys Ther 1998;27: 276–84.
20. Beumer A, Swierstra BA, Mulder PG. Clinical diagnosis of syndesmotic ankle instability: evaluation of stress tests behind the curtains. Acta Orthop Scand 2002;73:667–9.
21. Nussbaum ED, Hosea TM, Sieler SD, et al. Prospective evaluation of syndesmotic ankle sprains without diastasis. Am J Sports Med 2001;29:31–5.
22. Mabee J, Mabee C. Acute lateral sprained ankle syndrome. Internet J Fam Pract 2008;7.
23. Croy T, Koppenhaver S, Saliba S, et al. Anterior talocrural joint laxity: diagnostic accuracy of the anterior drawer test of the ankle. J Orthop Sports Phys Ther 2013; 43:911–9.
24. Fujii T, Luo ZP, Kitaoka HB, et al. The manual stress test may not be sufficient to differentiate ankle ligament injuries. Clin Biomech (Bristol, Avon) 2000;15: 619–23.
25. Kirk T, Saha S, Bowman LS. A new ankle laxity tester and its use in the measurement of the effectiveness of taping. Med Eng Phys 2000;22:723–31.
26. Lahde S, Putkonen M, Puranen J, et al. Examination of the sprained ankle: anterior drawer test or arthrography? Eur J Radiol 1988;8:255–7.
27. Maquirriain J. Achilles tendon rupture: avoiding tendon lengthening during surgical repair and rehabilitation. Yale J Biol Med 2011;84:289–300.
28. Simmonds FA. The diagnosis of the ruptured Achilles tendon. Practitioner 1957; 179:56–8.
29. Thompson TC. A test for rupture of the tendo Achilles. Acta Orthop Scand 1962; 32:461–5.
30. Cary DV. How to diagnose and manage an acute Achilles tendon rupture. JAAPA 2009;22:39–43.
31. Dowling S, Spooner CH, Liang Y, et al. Accuracy of Ottawa ankle rules to exclude fractures of the ankle and midfoot in children: a meta-analysis. Acad Emerg Med 2009;16:277–87.
32. Tayeb R. Diagnostic value of Ottawa ankle rules: simple guidelines with high sensitivity. Br J Sports Med 2013;47:e3, 28–9.
33. Glas AS, Pijnenburg BA, Lijmer JG, et al. Comparison of diagnostic decision rules and structured data collection in assessment of acute ankle injury. CMAJ 2002; 166:727–33.
34. Kievit JV, Dijkgraaf PB, Zwetsloot-Schonk JH, et al, Academic Hospital Leiden—Central Steering Institute. Steering of care, quality and information. Results and conclusions of two changes in the care process. Utrecht (Netherlands): Nationaal Ziekenhuis Instituut; 1991. p. 19–35.

35. Chinn L, Hertel J. Rehabilitation of ankle and foot injuries in athletes. Clin Sports Med 2010;29:157–67.
36. Wilken J, Rao S, Estin M, et al. A new device for assessing ankle dorsiflexion motion: reliability and validity. J Orthop Sports Phys Ther 2011;41:274–80.
37. Gould SJ, Cardone DA, Munyak J, et al. Sideline coverage: when to get radiographs? A review of clinical decision tools. Sports Health 2014;6:274–8.
38. Baravarian B, Thompson J, Nazarian D. Plantar plate tears: a review of the modified flexor tendon transfer repair for stabilization. Clin Podiatr Med Surg 2011;28: 57–68.
39. Creighton DW, Shrier I, Shultz R, et al. Return-to-play in sport: a decision-based model. Clin J Sport Med 2010;20:379–85.
40. Matheson GO, Shultz R, Bido J, et al. Return-to-play decisions: are they the team physician's responsibility? Clin J Sport Med 2011;21:25–30.
41. Petersen W, Zantop T. Return to play following ACL reconstruction: survey among experienced arthroscopic surgeons (AGA instructors). Arch Orthop Trauma Surg 2013;133:969–77.
42. Kaeding CC, Yu JR, Wright R, et al. Management and return to play of stress fractures. Clin J Sport Med 2005;15:442–7.

Acute Forefoot and Midfoot Injuries

R. Clinton Laird, DPM, FAAPSM, FACFAS

KEYWORDS

- Runner's toe • First metatarsal phalangeal joint dislocation
- Compartment syndrome • Jones fracture • Midfoot sprains
- Lisfranc fracture/dislocation

KEY POINTS

- Compartment syndrome and Lisfranc fractures require a high index of suspicion, because they both require further testing for accurate diagnosis.
- Fifth metatarsal base fractures must be examined closely, because treatment ranges from protected weight-bearing to surgical intervention.
- Radiographs of the first metatarsophalangeal joint dislocation must be evaluated closely to determine extent of damage.

SUBUNGUAL HEMATOMA

Subungual hematomas, commonly referred to as "runner's toe," are common injuries in runners. They are collections of blood under the nail plate. They cause intense pain and throbbing as pressure increases under the toenail. Runner's toe is caused by direct trauma to the nail, such as a crush injury (eg, dropping a heavy object on the nail) or, more commonly in running, microtrauma from rubbing on the end of a shoe. Shoe trauma can result from wearing a shoe that is too short or from normal swelling that occurs during high-mileage running. Another cause can be downhill running, wherein the foot slides forward in the shoe. Treatment ranges from none to surgical avulsion, depending on pain, and treatment of possible infection that can develop.

DIGITAL FRACTURES

Digital fractures are almost always a result of direct trauma. They are rarely debilitating but may require treatment and moderation of activity. Radiographs are required to determine treatment course. Treatment consists of rest, splinting to keep the toe in proper alignment, wearing of a stiff-soled shoe, "buddy splinting" if appropriate, and possible surgery to correct displacement with internal fixation. The formulation

Disclosure: The author has no financial disclosure to report.
17835 Murdock Circle Unit B, Port Charlotte, FL 33948, USA
E-mail address: footdr97@verizon.net

Clin Podiatr Med Surg 32 (2015) 231–238
http://dx.doi.org/10.1016/j.cpm.2014.11.005
podiatric.theclinics.com

of an alternative training schedule for athletes training for an event is important to prevent frustration and noncompliance.

METATARSAL FRACTURES

Metatarsal fractures represent 5% to 6% of fractures encountered in primary care.[1,2] These fractures range from requiring little treatment to requiring surgical intervention, depending on the location and displacement. Metatarsal fractures generally arise from direct trauma or twisting injuries.

Distal central metatarsal fractures (ie, neck fractures) are stable fractures and can be treated conservatively with a stiff-soled shoe or a walking fracture boot as long as there is less than 10° of sagittal plane deformity or greater than 4 mm translation. In those instances, percutaneous fixation should be considered with non–weight-bearing (NWB) casting.

First metatarsal fractures are more serious because of the weight-bearing (WB) forces they experience. If no displacement is present, limited WB in a fracture walking boot is acceptable treatment. If any displacement is present, surgery is indicated followed by NWB casting.

Fifth metatarsal fractures are the most common metatarsal fracture. Spiral oblique fractures (ie, Dancer's fractures) result from missteps and falls from the demi pointe position. The fracture is usually displaced and mildly comminuted. These fractures usually heal in a short leg cast for 6 to 8 weeks NWB. If it is significantly displaced, open reduction internal fixation (ORIF) may be required. Proximal fractures at the base of the fifth metatarsal are more difficult to treat. Fractures of the proximal fifth metatarsal are common and usually can be divided into 1 of 3 patterns:

- Avulsion fractures of the base of the metatarsal
- Fractures at the junction of the metaphysis and diaphysis (Jones fractures)
- Pure diaphysis fractures

Most of these fractures heal with nonoperative management and do not require surgery. Fractures of the metaphyseal diaphysis junction have a higher rate of nonunion and occasionally do require surgery. Jones fractures treated operatively have been shown to have excellent union rates.[3] Blood supply plays a crucial role in the healing ability of these fractures. As described by Smith and colleagues,[4] perfusion comes from metaphyseal arteries at the base of the fifth metatarsal. A nutrient artery enters at the proximal diaphysis and tracks proximally across the so-called "watershed area" at the metaphysis-diaphysis junction. This area creates a region at high risk for avascularity and poor healing with disruption of the blood supply. The Torg classification of fifth metatarsal base fractures (**Fig. 1**)[5] is as follows:

- Type 1: tuberosity fracture of the lateral aspect of the tuberosity extending proximally into the metatarsocuboid joint.
- Type 2: Jones fracture beginning laterally in the distal part of the tuberosity and extending obliquely and proximally into the medial cortex at the junction of the metaphysis and diaphysis.
- Type 3: fracture distal to the fourth and fifth metatarsal base articulation in the diaphyseal part of the bone.

Torg type I fractures can be treated in a removable fracture boot partial WB to full WB for 6 to 8 weeks. Torg types 2 and 3 fractures have been reported to have higher rates of nonunion treated nonoperatively than when treated surgically. The literature

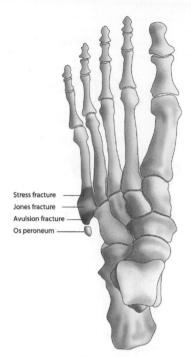

Stress fracture
Jones fracture
Avulsion fracture
Os peroneum

Fig. 1. Torg classification of fifth metatarsal base fractures. (*Reproduced* with permission from Dr Frank Gaillard, radiopaedia.org.)

supports early surgical treatment of type 2 and 3 fractures in performance athletes and of type 3 fractures with evidence of delayed union or nonhealing stress fractures.[6]

FIRST METATARSOPHALANGEAL JOINT INJURIES

The first metatarsophalangeal joint (MPJ) is frequently injured during sporting activities because of its higher range of motion and increased WB forces compared with the lesser MPJs.

"Turf toe" is an MPJ sprain representing an injury to the connective tissue between the foot and the hallux.[7,8] It occurs more commonly on harder surfaces, such as artificial turf; hence the name "turf toe." This injury can also occur in the lesser toes, and has been observed in participants of sports beyond American football, including soccer, basketball, rugby, volleyball, and tae kwon do.[9] Treatment involves limiting range of motion of the joint and rest. Taping and rigid inserts can be used to limit motion.

"Sand toe" injuries are plantarflexion injuries to the first MPJ that can lead to significant functional disability. A retrospective study by Frey and colleagues[10] reported that the average volleyball player took 6 months to heal. Conservative therapy should include taping, anti-inflammatory medications, shoewear modification, ice, and rest.

The Jahss classification for dislocation of the first MPJ is used to describe the high-energy hyperextension injuries that produce dislocation. Jahss[11] described first MPJ dislocation according to the involvement of the plantar plate and sesamoid complex. The Jahss classification (**Fig. 2**) is as follows:

- Type I: hallux dislocates and the intersesamoidal ligament is intact, necessitates surgical intervention.

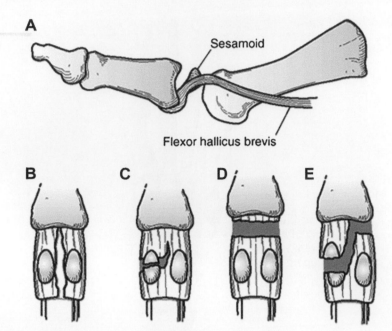

Fig. 2. Jahss classification of first MPJ dislocations. (*From* Jahss SA. Fractures of the proximal phalanges. A new method of reduction and immobilization. J Bone Joint Surg Am 1938;20:178–86; with permission.)

- Type IIA: intersesamoidal ligament is disrupted and the sesamoids diverge medially or laterally.
- Type IIB: intersesamoidal ligament is disrupted and a transverse sesamoid fracture is present.

Other authors subsequently added more types of first MPJ dislocations (IA, IB, IIC, III) to describe additional combinations.[12]

COMPARTMENT SYNDROME OF THE FOOT

Compartment syndrome occurs when excessive pressure builds up inside an enclosed space in the body, and usually results from bleeding or swelling after an injury. Compartment syndrome should be divided into 2 clinical entities. First, and most important, is acute compartment syndrome (ACS). The second, and still very important to the sports medicine physician, is chronic exertional compartment syndrome (CECS).

ACS occurs frequently after fractures or the treatment of those fractures (casting or surgical intervention). Other causes of ACS include crush injuries, burns, and blood clots in a vessel.

CECS usually develops over time as a result of muscle development and adaptation. The muscles hypertrophy because of prolonged exercise in an inelastic space (compartment).

Symptoms of compartment syndrome include the 6 Ps: pain out of proportion to what is expected based on the physical examination findings, paresthesia, pallor, paralysis, pulselessness, and poikilothermia. The first signs of compartment syndrome are numbness, tingling, and paresthesia.[13,14] Loss of function and decreased pulses or pulselessness, however, are late signs. Various recommendations for the intracompartmental pressure are used for diagnosis, with some sources quoting greater than 30 mm Hg[14] as an indication for fasciotomy, whereas others suggest that a less than 30 mm Hg difference between intracompartmental pressure and diastolic blood pressure warrants this procedure.[15] Various methods exist for measuring intracompartmental pressure, the most common of which is the Stryker Intra-Compartmental Pressure Monitor (Kalamazoo, MI, USA). Treatment for both ACS and CECS is fasciotomy of the compartments involved.

TENDON INJURIES OF THE MIDFOOT AND FOREFOOT

Acute tendon tears of the midfoot and forefoot are not common. These injuries can occur when the foot is in a fixed position and the tendon actively contracts and no motion occurs or from sharp trauma over the dorsum of the foot. Acute injuries can also occur with hyperflexion or extension injuries at the MPJs. Acute injuries can usually be diagnosed with proper physical examination, but may require advanced imaging techniques. Diagnostic ultrasound and MRI imaging can be useful in diagnosing minor tendon injuries.

Because of their superficial nature, the dorsal extensor tendons are subject to lacerations from objects falling on the top of the foot. Tendon lacerations can even occur without breaks in the skin. Acute rupture or laceration of a tendon requires surgical intervention and a NWB postoperative course.

MIDFOOT INJURIES

Midfoot sprains occur when an athlete sustains a twisting injury to the lower leg with the foot in a fixed position. All of the forces that should move with the foot on a yielding surface are transmitted through the foot, causing soft tissue damage. Many different athletes are subject to midfoot sprains, such as jockeys, windsurfers, football players, soccer players, basketball players, and field hockey players. Midfoot sprains were graded by Burroughs and colleagues (**Fig. 3**)[16]:

- Grade I: the injury is fairly mild, causing microscopic tears or stretching of the ligaments.
- Grade II (moderate): the ligaments may be partially torn, and the stretching is more severe.
- Grade III (severe): the ligaments are completely torn, and therefore the foot may be unstable and no longer able to bear weight.

Radiographs of these injuries should be taken while WB, if at all possible, to determine whether any separation occurred between the bones of the tarsometatarsal joint. If more significant injury is suspected, MRI should be obtained to evaluate the ligamentous structures and the osseous structures. Treatment for midfoot sprains ranges from rest to protected WB in a removable fracture boot.

LISFRANC FRACTURE DISLOCATION

Lisfranc fracture/dislocation injuries result if bones in the midfoot are broken or ligaments that support the midfoot are torn. The severity of the injury can vary from simple to complex, involving many joints and bones in the midfoot. Direct Lisfranc injuries are usually caused by a crush injury, such as a heavy object falling onto the midfoot, the foot being run over by a car or truck, or someone landing on the foot after a fall from a significant height.[17] In athletic trauma, Lisfranc injuries occur commonly in activities, such as windsurfing, kitesurfing, wakeboarding, or snowboarding (when appliance

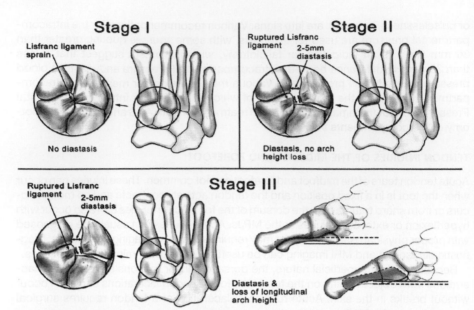

Fig. 3. Burroughs midfoot sprain classification. (*From* Nunley JA, Vertullo CJ. Classification, investigation, and management of midfoot sprains: Lisfranc injuries in the athlete. Am J Sports Med 2002;30(6):871–8; with permission.)

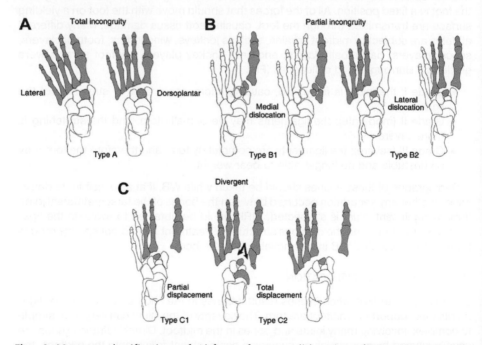

Fig. 4. Myerson classification of Lisfranc fracture dislocation. (*From* Myerson MS, Fisher RT, Burgess AR, et al. Fracture dislocations of the tarsometatarsal joints: end results correlated with pathology and treatment. Foot Ankle 1986;6(5):225–42; with permission.)

bindings pass directly over the metatarsals).[18] American football players occasionally acquire this injury, and it most often occurs when the athlete's foot is plantar flexed and another player lands on the heel. This injury can also occur during pivoting athletic positions, such as performed by a baseball catcher or a ballerina spinning. Typically these patients will be unable to bear weight. Radiographs should show bony abnormality. If plain films are not definitive, MRI or computed tomography scan should be obtained if a high index of suspicion exists. Myerson and colleagues[19] classified Lisfranc fracture dislocations into different types (**Fig. 4**):

- Total incongruity: medial or lateral
- Partial incongruity: B1 medial or B2 lateral (most common)
- Divergent displacement: C1 partial or C2 total

Treatment for Lisfranc fracture dislocations can include nonoperative and operative courses. If the dislocation is less than 2 mm, NWB casting for 6 weeks can be used. For more significant dislocations, ORIF with K-wires or temporary screws with 6 weeks NWB followed by hardware removal and protected WB is the usual treatment course.

REFERENCES

1. Hatch RL, Rosenbaum CI. Fracture care by family physicians. A review of 295 cases. J Fam Pract 1994;38:238–44.
2. Eiff MP, Saultz JW. Fracture care by family physicians. J Am Board Fam Pract 1993;6:179–81.
3. Clapper MF, O'Brien TJ, Lyons PM. Fractures of the fifth metatarsal: analysis of a fracture registry. Clin Orthop Relat Res 1995;315:238–41.
4. Smith JW, Arnoczky SP, Hersh A. The intraosseous blood supply of the fifth metatarsal: implications for proximal fracture healing. Foot Ankle 1992;13:143–52.
5. Hartog BD. Fractures of the proximal fifth metatarsal. J Am Acad Orthop Surg 2009;17(7):458–64.
6. Kelly IP, Glisson RR, Fink C, et al. Intramedullary screw fixation of Jones fractures. Foot Ankle Int 2001;22:585–9.
7. Allen LR, Flemming D, Sanders TG. Turf toe: ligamentous injury of the first metatarsophalangeal joint. Mil Med 2004;169(11):xix–xxiv.
8. Kubitz ER. Athletic injuries of the first metatarsophalangeal joint. J Am Podiatr Med Assoc 2003;93(4):325–32.
9. Frimenko RE, Lievers W, Coughlin MJ, et al. Etiology and biomechanics of first metatarsophalangeal joint sprains (turf toe) in athletes. Crit Rev Biomed Eng 2012;40(1):43–61.
10. Frey C, Andersen GD, Feder KS. Plantarflexion injury to the metatarsophalangeal joint ("sand toe"). Foot Ankle Int 1996;17(9):576–81.
11. Jahss SA. Fractures of the proximal phalanges. A new method of reduction and immobilization. J Bone Joint Surg Am 1938;20:178–86.
12. Packer GJ, Shakeen MA. Patterns of hand fractures and dislocations in a district general hospital. J Hand Surg Br 1993;18:511–4.
13. Compartment syndrome: fractures, dislocations, and sprains. Merck Manual Professional.
14. Emedicine: compartment syndrome.
15. Pocketbook of orthopaedics and fractures: Ronald McRae.
16. Burroughs KE, Reimer CD, Fields KB. Lisfranc injury of the foot: a commonly missed diagnosis. Am Fam Physician 1998;58(1):118–24.

17. Chan SC, Chow SP. Current concept review on Lisfranc injuries. J Orthop Surg (Hong Kong) 2001;5(1):75–80.
18. Lievers WB, Frimenko RE, Crandall JR, et al. Age, sex, causal and injury patterns in tarsometatarsal dislocations: a literature review of over 2000 cases. Foot (Edinb) 2012;22(3):117–24.
19. Myerson MS, Fisher RT, Burgess AR, et al. Fracture dislocation of the tarsometatarsal joints: end results correlated with pathology and treatment. Foot Ankle 1986;6(5):225–42.

Overuse Lower Extremity Injuries in Sports

Brian W. Fullem, DPM

KEYWORDS

- Medial tibial stress syndrome • Achilles tendonopathy • Iliotibial band syndrome
- Stress fractures • Eccentric strengthening • Core strength

KEY POINTS

- Medial tibial stress syndrome is a common overuse injury, particularly in new runners. Diagnostically one must differentiate between a stress fracture and soft tissue injury. Treatment may include a relative rest period, and athletes are encouraged to participate in cross-training. Strengthening and sport-specific training are imperative before return to activity.
- ITBS is most common in distance runners and cyclists. Stretching plays a part in the treatment but it has been proved that strengthening of the core muscles, in particular the hip abductors, is the most important aspect of treatment.
- Stress fractures typically present with an insidious onset and pain increasing as the activity progresses. Radiograph should only be considered an initial screening tool and a negative result is not conclusive as far as a fracture is concerned. MRI, CT scan, and bone scintography should all be used to make a proper diagnosis.
- A sports medicine professional has an obligation to make a diagnosis and treat the cause of the injury to safely return the athlete to their respective sport.

INTRODUCTION

Physical fitness has become an important lifestyle choice for a portion of the population. When athletes train harder, the risk of injury increases. This article explores several common overuse injuries to the lower extremity including medial tibial stress syndrome (MTSS), iliotibial band syndrome (ITBS), and stress fractures. Many articles[1-3] have shown that these are among the most commonly diagnosed lower limb injuries caused by overuse. Our charge as sports medicine professionals is to identify and treat the cause of the injuries and not just treat the symptoms. Symptomatology is an excellent guide to healing and often the patient leads the physician to the proper

Disclosure: None.
Private Practice: Elite Sports Podiatry, 1700 North McMullen Booth Road, C-2, Clearwater, FL 33759, USA
E-mail address: DoctorFullem@gmail.com

Clin Podiatr Med Surg 32 (2015) 239–251
http://dx.doi.org/10.1016/j.cpm.2014.11.006   **podiatric.theclinics.com**

diagnosis through an investigation of the athlete's training program, past injury history, dietary habits, choice of footwear, and training surface.

MEDIAL TIBIAL STRESS SYNDROME

MTSS in layman's terms is often referred to as "shin splints." It is a more common complaint for the novice athlete. There are several differential diagnoses that fall under this term but most commonly the athlete is experiencing MTSS. There are often intrinsic and extrinsic factors causing this injury including gastrocnemius-soleus tightness, deep posterior muscle group weakness, tibial varum, improper biomechanics, training on hard surfaces, training errors, and worn-out running shoes.

To date, there is a lack of high-quality level one evidence studies on the subject. In a recent article Hamstra-Wright and coworkers[4] state "There is a need for high-quality, prospective studies using consistent methodology evaluating MTSS risk factors." Newman and colleagues[5] published a meta-analysis of the last 40 years on risk factors for MTSS and found that it affects 5% to 35% of runners and includes a prior history of the injury, increased body mass index, increased navicular drop, and increased external hip rotation in males to all be factors but the causative factors remain inconclusive. Yuksel and colleagues[6] found that some athletes with MTSS have an imbalance of inverters and everters of the foot and ankle. Strengthening these groups of muscles was shown to be helpful. Note that the strengthening exercises to follow in the IT band portion are also applicable for MTSS.

These patients typically exhibit more pain at the start of a run. Although it subsides during the run, the patient then has more pain after stopping. MTSS pain occurs along the lower third of the posterior medial surface of the tibia, which coincides with the origin of the posterior tibial muscle and the soleus muscle.[7] Yates and Bennett found that a pronated foot type was statistically significant for predicting MTSS to occur in naval recruits and high school runners, respectively.[8–10] In chronic cases of MTSS, one notes pain with palpation along a diffuse portion of the medial tibia and palpable scar tissue.

Treating Medial Tibal Stress Syndrome

There are different phases to the treatment of MTSS. The first phase is aimed at reducing pain and inflammation. Relative rest is required during this phase but one can allow cross-training as long as it does not increase any of the symptoms. Biking, swimming, the elliptical trainer, and pool running are all excellent ways to maintain aerobic fitness. One should use physical therapy modalities, deep tissue massage, stretching, ice massage with frozen paper cups, and/or the Alter G treadmill.

Shockwave therapy when compared with a control group was found to allow runners to return to activity in 59 days versus 91 days.[11] Shock-absorbing insoles, strengthening including the core muscles, and a gradual return to training have all proved to be effective at reducing symptoms and faster return to activity.[11–13]

The next phase involves the introduction of strength and proprioception training as tolerated while the patient maintains many of the tasks he or she initiated in phase one. Once the patient is pain-free and can perform isometric and isotonic strengthening exercises with no pain, he or she can then start the final phase, which involves eccentric and plyometric exercises aimed at strengthening the muscles in the way that they are used during running. Jumping on a mini-trampoline and jumping rope are two excellent plyometric type exercises that help to strengthen the posterior muscle groups that become weakened during MTSS.

A well-constructed orthotic device with shock absorption may be another part of the treatment plan. A varus ethylene vinyl acetate forefoot post extending to the sulcus in a pronated foot type often helps to reduce the symptoms of MTSS and addresses navicular drop as a possible causative factor.[5]

These patients should perform daily barefoot exercises to maintain strength and function of the intrinsic musculature after they start using orthotic devices. One exercise I often advise my patients to perform is to balance on each foot for 1 minute every time they brush their teeth. When their proprioception improves, they can do this with their eyes closed to make it more challenging. Patients can start running every other day. They should start initially on softer surfaces with no more than a 10% increase in mileage per week until they reach preinjury training levels. A study by Nielsen and colleagues[6] examined novice runners and found that those increasing their mileage by 10% per week or less had fewer injuries.

ILIOTIBIAL BAND SYNDROME

ITBS remains one of the main causes of knee pain in runners and also occurs commonly in cyclists. It is unique to these two sports because of the repetitive nature of performing the same exercise mainly in one plane of motion for extended periods of time. ITBS was not identified in the literature until 1975 by Renne.[14]

The Ilitotibial band is a fibrous structure that serves to assist the stability of the leg during stance phase (the period of time that the foot is in contact with the ground) and helps to resist torsional movements around the knee joint. The IT band begins in the hip as the tensor fascia lata muscle and ends below the knee joint inserting into the tibia at a landmark known as Gerdy tubercle. The most common location of pain is the lateral femoral condyle on the side of the knee before the ITB crosses the knee joint to end at the insertion point. The pain usually presents itself just after heel contact and is aggravated by the length of time that one is running and may progressively get worse as the run progresses. Downhill and long slow running are two factors that tend to cause an increase in symptoms (**Fig. 1**).

Fredericson at Stanford University discovered that weakness of the hip abductor muscles (which consist mainly of the gluteus minimus and gluteus medius) was the leading cause of ITBS. He reported[15] on the cause of ITBS and developed a treatment plan that remains the gold standard of treatment. Research in the interim has only served to prove Fredericson was correct in his original assumptions. In 2007, Noehren and colleagues[16] reported that after studying the three-dimensional kinematics of female runners, that those who develop ITBS have an increased hip abduction along with greater knee internal rotation, both findings thought to be caused by weakness in the hip abductors.

One can assess the strength of the hip with some simple tests. Analysis by a sports medicine professional can usually identify any weakness or tightness of the involved structures (**Fig. 2**). A hip drop typically occurs when one foot is in contact with the ground if there is a weakness. Ideally runners should have the hips remain level throughout the gait cycle. The hip of the leg not in contact with the ground drops and this is known as a positive Trendelenburg sign and is an indicator that the opposite hip is weaker. This leads to increase stress on the side that is in the stance phase (**Fig. 3**).

Fredericson divides the treatment of this injury into three phases. The initial phase centers on reducing the pain and inflammation and increasing the mobilization of the IT band. Ice, rest, nonsteroidal anti-inflammatory drugs, topical anti-inflammatory drugs, and occasionally a corticosteroid injection can all be used to

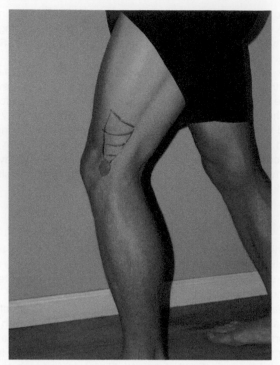

Fig. 1. The distal aspect of the IT band is highlighted with the common area of pain in red at the lateral femoral condyle.

help in this initial phase. Corticosteroid injections are commonly afforded a bad reputation but in this case it is an excellent choice to reduce the pain and enable one to move onto the next phase of treatment when used judiciously, with the understanding that the injection is not curing the injury. Deep tissue massage is another important part of the treatment in this phase and can be performed solo with the use of a foam roller **(Fig. 4)**.

Stretching **(Fig. 5)** can then be added and deep tissue massage should be continued to mobilize the tissue and prepare the leg to be strengthened. Training can be resumed when the pain level is reduced enough so that there is not any limping

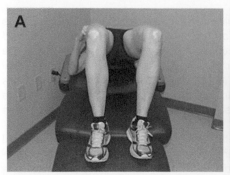
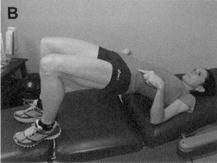

Fig. 2. (*A, B*) Hips should remain level when you bridge up from the table.

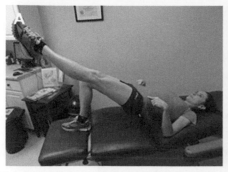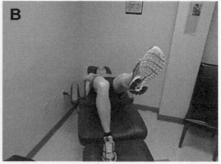

Fig. 3. (*A, B*) A more advanced method of checking hip abductor strength. Leg is extended to help assess weakness and is also a good strengthening exercise.

or compensation. Strides can sometimes be performed early in the treatment phase because it has been found that shorter and faster running does not make the injury worse.

Strengthening can be initiated when the exercises can be performed painlessly. If one has access to an Alter G treadmill that may also allow continued running during the rehabilitation phase. This treadmill can allow as little as 10% of body weight to impact the treadmill; a pressurized vacuum is created after zipping special neoprene shorts into the device (**Fig. 6**).

One can begin strengthening by using an elastic therapy band to perform a clam-shell exercise. The exercise should be performed slowly with emphasis on good form. Try to build up to 10 repetitions of three sets of each exercise. When this exercise becomes easier and the leg remains pain free during the exercises one can move on to more advanced strengthening (**Fig. 7**).

Side leg lifts are highlighted in **Fig. 8**: perform 10 repetitions of each leg and build up to three sets. Form is very important. The top hip needs to be in front of the body or anterior and the sequence should be performed slowly with toe pointed down. Raise leg straight up, then back, then forward and then back down to starting position. Build up to three sets of 10 repetitions.

Single-leg one-quarter squats are another excellent exercise to perform. It is impor-tant that the leg goes straight over the foot (**Fig. 9**).

These exercises can then be made more challenging by mimicking running form initially and then moving further by touching the ground out in front of the body

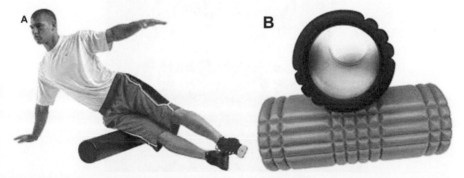

Fig. 4. (*A, B*) A type of foam roller and use for self-massage.

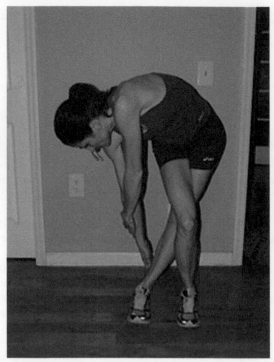

Fig. 5. The most effective stretch for ITBS according to Fredericson and coworkers.[17] Left leg is being stretched, hold the pose for 15 seconds and repeat 10 times, perform three sets a day.

(**Fig. 10**). Next a ball can used moving it up and down diagonally and then side to side in a twisting motion (**Fig. 11**).

Eccentric strengthening is one of the final exercises to be performed and helps to strengthen the hip abductors in the same manner in which they function during running. Hip hikes can be performed on a step stool as shown in **Fig. 12**A or on the stairs. Perform 10 repetitions on each side and build up to three sets.

One can test the injured leg with short runs that can be extended as long as the pain is not causing a limp or any compensation. It is difficult to place a time frame for

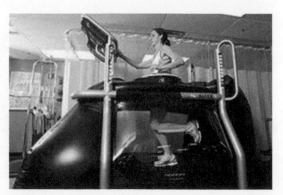

Fig. 6. Alter G treadmill.

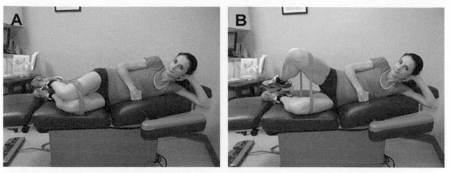

Fig. 7. (*A, B*) Clam shell strengthening exercise with an elastic therapy band.

recovery because such factors as how long the leg has been injured and other biomechanical factors may lengthen the recovery process. If the foot overpronates then a visit to a sports podiatrist is imperative to possibly consider custom foot orthoses, but keep in mind that those without significant pronation may actually get increased symptoms if one controls too much of the pronatory motion of the foot. The ideal treatment plan can sometimes include input from podiatrists, physical medicine specialists and physical therapists, chiropractors, or orthopedists.

STRESS FRACTURES

The treatment of stress fractures in athletes can be a challenging task especially when treating athletes who are competing in school, professionally, or at the highest

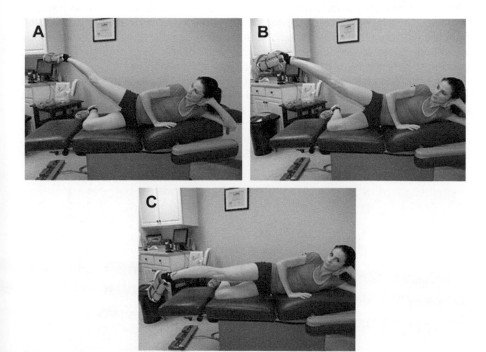

Fig. 8. (*A–C*) Side leg lifts.

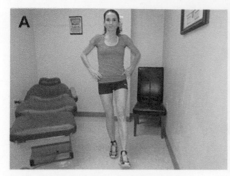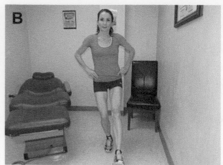

Fig. 9. (*A, B*) One-quarter leg squat.

recreational levels. These athletes often have a narrow time frame to train and compete in their desired sporting activities. Reducing healing time by every means possible is crucial to the success of these athletes and, in turn, achieving success as a sports medicine physician.

In 1855, Breithaupt[18] first described stress fractures as "march fractures" and made the clinical description of swelling and pain in the foot of a metatarsal stress fracture. The fractures were closely associated with the marching of soldiers.

Matheson and colleagues[19] analyzed cases of 320 athletes with bone scan–positive stress fractures treated over 3.5 years and assessed the results of conservative management. The most common bone injured was the tibia (49.1%), followed by the tarsals (25.3%), metatarsals (8.8%), femur (7.2%), fibula (6.6%), pelvis (1.6%), sesamoids (0.9%), and spine (0.6%). Stress fractures were bilateral in 16.6% of cases.

The literature often points to overuse as one of the main causes of a stress fracture. Overuse or training errors can account for the extrinsic factors in an injury. However, there are typically other more intrinsic factors, such as poor bone density, low body weight, weakness of the core muscles, and biomechanical abnormalities including limb length differences, all of which can lead to a stress fracture.

Fredericson and colleagues[20] found that athletes who played ball sports, such as basketball or soccer, during childhood had a decreased incidence of stress fractures as adults. One can make a correlation that these athletes have developed better core musculature particularly their hip abductors, which leads to fewer injuries.

Akuthota and colleagues[21] have further proved that improving hip abductor strength is the key component for treatment of ITBS.[22] They note that improving hip abductor

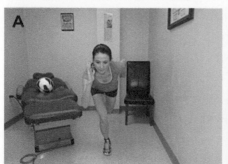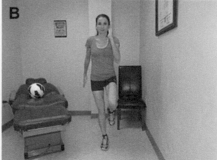

Fig. 10. (*A, B*) More advanced one-quarter squat.

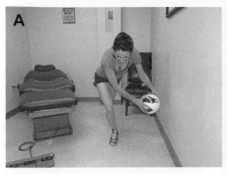
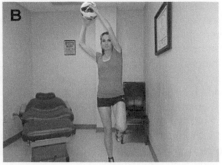

Fig. 11. (*A, B*) Core strengthening using a soccer ball.

strength is also useful in the prevention and treatment of other lower extremity injuries, such as Achilles tendonitis and MTSS.[21,22] Athletes are often searching for ways to improve performance and adding a core strengthening program is arguably the best way to help prevent injury leading to improved performance.

Diagnosis of Stress Fractures

To diagnose and treat stress fractures effectively, one must have a high index of suspicion during the initial clinical examination. Stress fractures are often accompanied by increased pain as the activity or workout progresses. This is the opposite of soft tissue injuries, which typically hurt more at the start.

One diagnostic test that works well is having the patient hop on the injured side. This produces sharp, pinpoint pain. One may also use the hop test to determine if the bone is healed enough for the patient to return to activity.

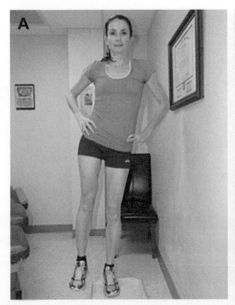
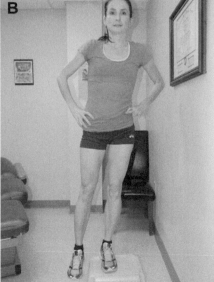

Fig. 12. (*A, B*) Hip hikes, which strengthen the hip abductors in an eccentric manner.

Most physicians have radiographs readily available, and with the advent of digital X-ray equipment it is sometimes possible to pick up a stress fracture earlier than ever. One must keep in mind that negative radiographs should almost never rule out a stress fracture. Some bones, such as the navicular or cuboid, may never exhibit radiographic changes in the presence of a stress fracture. Although metatarsal stress fractures can sometimes be seen on radiograph, it is typically at the point where the bone has healed and symptoms have subsided that there is radiographic evidence of bone healing (see **Fig. 12B**; **Fig. 13**).

If initial radiographs are negative and further testing is required, then the physician can choose between MRI, Tc99 bone scintigraphy, and computed tomography (CT) scanning. There is some debate as to whether MRI or bone scan is better for diagnosing a stress fracture.

Dobrindt and colleagues[23] recently published an article supporting the use of bone scintigraphy. Three different observers studied bone scans without any clinical information about the patient for the diagnosis of stress injuries in 50 of 93 patients. Researchers found that the mean sensitivity, specificity, positive predictive value, negative predictive value, and accuracy were 97.3%, 67.4%, 77.7%, 95.6%, and 83.5%, respectively. An analysis showed a high agreement among the three different observers.

Research has shown MRI to have a higher specificity for detecting the exact location for the injury. However, one must use caution in interpreting MRI results because bone marrow edema, which is commonly associated with a stress reaction or stress fracture, can also be seen in asymptomatic individuals.

A CT scan is a much better option for some bones, such as the navicular or cuboid, and when an MRI is inconclusive, and shows an increase of bone marrow edema. CT shows the cortex of bone much better than MRI.

Takacs and coworkers[24] presented a case study of a patient with multiple stress fractures, who used the Alter G treadmill while rehabilitating from these fractures.

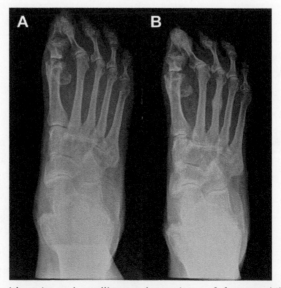

Fig. 13. Patient with pain and swelling and no signs of fracture (A). Patient almost asymptomatic for follow-up 1 month later and stress fracture healing evident (B).

The patient experienced a significant reduction in pain and an improvement in ankle range of motion, walking speed, and physical function, which the researchers assessed via the Foot and Ankle Module of the American Academy of Orthopedic Surgeons Lower Limb Outcomes Assessment Instrument. Training did not seem to have any adverse effect on fracture healing as was evident on the radiograph.

A good general rule of thumb to guide treatment is that patients should avoid anything that causes pain. Use of a surgical shoe to offload the painful area often suffices for metatarsal stress fractures. If the patient has pain when walking in a surgical shoe, then it may be necessary to move to a controlled ankle motion walker. If pain is still present, then nonweightbearing may be warranted. The addition of a high ankle brace can be helpful with tibial and fibular stress fractures.

Navicular stress fractures in particular occur in runners at a surprisingly high rate and require more aggressive conservative treatment. The Matheson study found that 25% of the fractures were of tarsal bones.[19] The diagnosis and treatment of navicular stress fractures require a high index of suspicion and 8 to 10 weeks of immobilization including nonweightbearing.

Bone Stimulation and Shockwave Therapy as Adjunctive Therapies

Bone stimulation may also help an injured athlete recover faster from a stress fracture. A study by Saxena[25] showed that using a pulsed electromagnetic field allowed athletes to return much quicker from their stress fractures. Saxena presented a small, prospective, unblinded analysis of 73 stress fractures that were confirmed via bone scan, MRI, or CT scan. The electromagnetic group returned to activity in 8.8 weeks versus the nonelectromagnetic group, which returned to activity in 17.6 weeks.

Uchiyama and colleagues[26] presented a study on the use of low-intensity pulsed ultrasound in the treatment of anterior tibial stress fractures. These fractures are notoriously slow to heal. One aspect of this study that differentiates it from other studies is the evaluation of the return to full activity for athletes, making it more applicable for sports medicine. Athletes returned to full activity two to three times faster with the use of bone stimulation in comparison with other modalities for the same injury.

Further scientific studies are warranted but returning to activity even a few weeks earlier can mean a great difference to a professional runner or a college or high school runner with a limited amount of eligibility to compete. The use of bone stimulation has almost no downside other than cost.

Extracorporeal shockwave therapy (ESWT) is another modality that shows promise to help improve healing times for stress fractures. Taki and colleagues[27] examined five athletes who had delayed or nonunions of stress fractures, and each injury showed significant improvements. The authors opined that ESWT promotes osteogenesis and helped these athletes heal faster.

Moretti and coworkers[28] also found that ESWT can speed the healing process. They conducted a retrospective study of 10 athletes affected by chronic stress fractures of the fifth metatarsal and tibia who received three to four sessions of low-middle energy ESWT. The authors concluded that at the follow-up (8 weeks on average), the clinical and radiography results were excellent, and enabled all players to gradually return to sports activities.

These reports show that ESWT is a noninvasive and effective treatment of resistant stress fractures. Similar to the use of bone stimulation, there are no known negative effects for the use of shockwave therapy for stress fractures.

REFERENCES

1. Yeung EW, Yeung SS. A systematic review of interventions to prevent lower limb soft tissue running injuries. Br J Sports Med 2001;35(6):383–9.
2. Heir T, Edie G. Age, body composition, aerobic fitness and health condition as risk factors for musculoskeletal injuries. Scand J Med Sci Sports 1996;6:222–7.
3. Vleck VE, Garbutt G. Injury and training characteristics of male elite, development squad, and club triathletes. Int J Sports Med 1998;19:38–42.
4. Hamstra-Wright KL, Huxel Bliven KC, Bay C. Risk factors for medial tibial stress syndrome in physically active individuals such as runners and military personnel: a systematic review and meta-analysis. Br J Sports Med 2014 [Epub ahead of print].
5. Newman P, Witchalls J, Waddington G, et al. Risk factors associated with medial tibial stress syndrome in runners: a systematic review and meta-analysis. Open Access J Sports Med 2013;4:229–41.
6. Yüksel O, Özgürbüz C, Ergün M, et al. Inversion/Eversion Strength Dysbalance in Patients With Medial Tibial Stress Syndrome. J Sports Sci Med 2011 December; 10(4):737–42. Published online December 1, 2011.
7. Saxena A, O'Brien T, Bunce D. Anatomic dissection of the tibialis posterior muscle and its correlation to medial tibial stress syndrome. J Foot Surg 1990;29(2): 105–8.
8. Yates B, White S. The incidence and risk factors in the development of medial tibial stress syndrome among naval recruits. Am J Sports Med 2004;32(3):772–80.
9. Bennett JE, Reinking MF, Pluemer B, et al. Factors contributing to the development of medial tibial stress syndrome in high school runners. J Orthop Sports Phys Ther 2001;31(9):504–10.
10. Bouche RT. Chronic compartment syndrome of the leg. J Am Podiatr Med Assoc 1990;80(12):633–48.
11. Moen MH, Rayer S, Schipper M, et al. Shockwave treatment for medial tibial stress syndrome in athletes; a prospective controlled study. Br J Sports Med 2012;46(4):253–7.
12. Rompe JD, Cacchio A, Furia JP, et al. Low-energy extracorporeal shock wave therapy as a treatment for medial tibial stress syndrome. Am J Sports Med 2010;38(1):125–32.
13. Reshef N, Guelich DR. Medial tibial stress syndrome. Clin Sports Med 2012; 31(2):273–90.
14. Renne JW. The iliotibial band friction syndrome. J Bone Joint Surg Am 1975; 57(8):1110–1.
15. Fredericson M, Cookingham CL, Chaudhari AM, et al. Hip abductor weakness in distance runners with iliotibial band syndrome. Clin J Sport Med 2000;10(3): 169–75.
16. Noehren B, Davis I, Hamill J. ASB clinical biomechanics award winner 2006 prospective study of the biomechanical factors associated with iliotibial band syndrome. Clin Biomech (Bristol, Avon) 2007;22(9):951–6.
17. Fredericson M, White JJ, Macmahon JM, et al. Quantitative analysis of the relative effectiveness of 3 iliotibial band stretches. Arch Phys Med Rehabil 2002;83(5): 589–92.
18. Breithaupt MD. Zur pathologie Des Mensch Lichen Fusses. Med Zeitung 1855; 24:169–71, 175–7.
19. Matheson GO, Clement DB, McKenzie DC, et al. Stress fractures in athletes. A study of 320 cases. Am J Sports Med 1987;15(1):46–58.

20. Fredericson M, Ngo J, Cobb K. Effects of ball sports on future risk of stress fracture in runners. Clin J Sport Med 2005;15(3):136–41.
21. Akuthota V, Ferreiro A, Moore T, et al. Core stability exercise principles. Curr Sports Med Rep 2008;7(1):39–44.
22. Fredericson M, Wolf C. Iliotibial band syndrome in runners: innovations in treatment. Sports Med 2005;35(5):451–9.
23. Dobrindt O, Hoffmeyer B, Ruf J, et al. Blinded-read of bone scintigraphy: the impact on diagnosis and healing time for stress injuries with emphasis on the foot. Clin Nucl Med 2011;36(3):186–91.
24. Takacs J, Leiter JR, Peeler JD. Novel application of lower body positive-pressure in the rehabilitation of an individual with multiple lower extremity fractures. J Rehabil Med 2011;43(7):653–6.
25. Saxena A. Treatment of lower extremity stress fractures with pulsed electromagnetic fields (PEMF): a case-control study and comparison to the literature. Foot Ankle Quarterly 2000;13(2):43–50.
26. Uchiyama Y, Nakamura Y, Mochida J, et al. Effect of low-intensity pulsed ultrasound treatment for delayed and non-union stress fractures of the anterior mid-tibia in five athletes. Tokai J Exp Clin Med 2007;32(4):121–5.
27. Taki M, Iwata O, Shiono M, et al. Extracorporeal shock wave therapy for resistant stress fracture in athletes: a report of 5 cases. Am J Sports Med 2007;35(7):1188–92.
28. Moretti B, Notarnicola A, Garofalo R, et al. Shock waves in the treatment of stress fractures. Ultrasound Med Biol 2009;35(6):1042–9.

Considerations in Treating Physically Active Older Adults and Aging Athletes

Paul R. Langer, DPM, ABPM, FAAPSM

KEYWORDS

• Aging • Exercise • Physical activity • Injuries • Successful aging

KEY POINTS

- There are significant physiologic and physical changes that occur with age. Appreciating these changes is important when treating older patients.
- Physical activity and exercise have many benefits in the older population. Improved cognitive function, physical well-being, and management of common chronic conditions are but some of the benefits that combine to significantly impact quality of life and offset natural declines associated with aging.
- Podiatrists can and should promote the benefits of exercise to their patients.

Medical practitioners learn in school not to treat children as "little adults" because there are so many physical and physiologic differences between an adult and a child but they also need to bear in mind that treating older adults is not the same as treating younger adults for precisely the same reasons. Understanding the physical and physiologic changes of aging is important so sports medicine practitioners can tailor treatment plans and patient education so as to best treat musculoskeletal injuries and to help minimize the risk of reinjury.

The US Public Health Service declared that exercise is 1 of the 5 priority areas to prevent premature morbidity and mortality. The National Council on Aging recommends that older adults "engage in moderate physical activity for at least 30 minutes 5 days a week and muscle-strengthening activities on 2 or more days a week that work all major muscle groups." However, statistics show that fewer than one-third of Americans aged 65 and older meet this level.[1] Medical professionals owe it to their patients to not only treat their current conditions but also to educate them on the benefits of maintaining or starting a fitness program so that they may enjoy a better quality of life as they age.

Although age-related changes are unavoidable, research is suggesting that many of the declines previously associated with aging may be actually more due to the

Disclosure: None.
4010 West 65th Street, Edina, MN 55435, USA
E-mail address: paullanger@tcomn.com

Clin Podiatr Med Surg 32 (2015) 253–260
http://dx.doi.org/10.1016/j.cpm.2014.11.007
0891-8422/15/$ – see front matter © 2015 Elsevier Inc. All rights reserved.

sedentary lifestyle that many older individuals adopt.[2,3] Some researchers estimate that exercise can offset the aging decline by up to 50%.[4–7] In addition to the natural aging process, many older individuals also have chronic diseases, such as hypertension, osteoarthritis, diabetes, or cardiac disease. Regular exercise has long been a recommended part of management for these conditions. Hessert and colleagues[8] published a study that showed that elders who participated in a functional fitness program made significant improvements in the fitness parameters studied. They combined exercises that addressed mobility, strength, balance, dexterity, and flexibility. They concluded that exercise was a good complement to older adults' other medical management strategies, such as pharmaceuticals, surgery, and nutrition.

Exercise is much more important than just a weight management tool. Its benefits go well beyond burning calories. This bodes well for older adults and provides an opportunity for medical practitioners to speak to their patients about the importance of remaining active or increasing physical activity as they age to maximize their health and quality of life.

Weight gain with aging is unfortunately common and of course exercise is important in managing weight. In fact, Montoye and colleagues[9] found that previously athletic individuals who stop participating in sport have a rapid weight gain beginning at age 45. Other studies show that even individuals who have previously been sedentary can significantly decrease their risk of serious illness and risk of disability by starting a fitness program later in life. The National Institute on Aging at the National Institutes of Health has a Web site and exercise program specifically for older individuals called go4life, which describes very well the benefits of exercise and provides detailed information on exercise programs.[10]

The volume of research on aging is increasingly showing that there are physical, cognitive, and psychosocial benefits to remaining physically active.[7,8,11–13] Older individuals are more prone to overuse injuries and are slower to heal than younger individuals for reasons that will be discussed later in this article. Despite the increased risk of injury, however, researchers and clinicians agree that the benefits of exercise far outweigh the risks.

The cognitive and neurologic benefits of physical activity are broad and just as important as the physical benefits. In older individuals, exercise improves learning and memory, and has both therapeutic and preventive effects on depression.[11] Research also has shown delayed onset and reduced risk of Alzheimer, Parkinson, and Huntington diseases in physically active individuals.[14–16]

Some research shows that the benefits of an active lifestyle may have payoffs later in life. Rovio and colleagues[17] found that leisure time physical activity at mid-life at least twice a week was associated with a reduced risk of dementia in individuals between the ages of 65 and 79.

There are a number of fitness activities that provide different health benefits and a well-rounded fitness routine should include different activities to maximize those benefits. One year of endurance training improved maximum oxygen uptake to the level of a sedentary person 10 to 20 years younger and also improved muscle function and decreased body fat.[18] A literature review on physical activity and aging suggests that it is important to combine endurance training with resistance training to reap the maximum benefit of exercise.[19]

AGE-RELATED PHYSICAL AND PHYSIOLOGIC CHANGES

The aging process starts earlier than many people suspect. Studies show that some physiologic and physical changes begin as early the third decade of life. This decline progresses in a linear fashion until approximately age 60 to 70 when there is a steeper drop-off.[20] Some of the important declines that occur that are significant in the older patient are discussed in the following sections.

Vascular Changes

Cardiac, vascular, and pulmonary functions decline at a rate of approximately 10% per decade after age 25.[21] Decreased maximal heart rate and myocardial contraction, increased peripheral vascular resistance, diminished lung capacity, and decreased alveolar gas exchange are just some of the changes that combine to decrease the delivery of oxygen to muscle and other soft tissue.[10] It is extremely important that all patients have a preactivity examination by a physician because underlying cardiac disease increases the risk of myocardial infarction and sudden cardiac death. For this reason, even fit patients should have regular follow-up examinations with their physician to monitor for changes that might alter their risk factors.[22]

Neurologic Changes

Neurologic changes include loss of nerve tissue, including cerebral cortex and spinal cord axons and dysfunction of peripheral nerves.[5] These losses affect not only cognition but also coordination, fine motor skills, proprioception, and balance. Dorfman and Bosley[23] found a 30% to 50% reduction in ankle proprioception and vibration sense in aged subjects. Depression and some medications also can have negative effects on neuromuscular coordination.[24] Impaired balance and worries about falling are 2 of the most often cited reasons for decreased activity in older individuals.[25] Addressing those fears and deficits in balance are important, as most acute injuries in older persons are related to falls or slips.[26,27] Research shows that training balance and lower extremity strength simultaneously is an important strategy in maintaining physical function and decreasing the risk of falls.[28,29]

Muscle Changes

There is a 20% to 40% decrease in strength between the ages of 20 and 70.[30,31] Age-related decline in muscle function is thought to have the greatest impact on functional capacity.[23] Sarcopenia describes the process of muscle deterioration, which includes reduced number and size of muscle cells and also includes decreased density of mitochondria. Sarcopenia results in decreased muscle power and endurance. Wolfson and colleagues[28] showed strength and balance improvements in older subjects with a laboratory-based training program. Their study subjects then transitioned to a Tai Chi program and were able to maintain the gains, although to a lesser degree. Unlike the muscle hypertrophy seen in younger individuals, improved motor unit recruitment seems to be the mechanism by which strength training provides a benefit in older individuals.[7] The preservation of muscle power into late life can greatly decrease the risk of disability and enhance functional independence.[32]

Tendon Changes

Aging itself is not a risk factor in tendon injuries, but changes to the cellular matrix of tendons occur with age.[33] Increased collagen, decreased collagen turnover, increased cross-linking, and changes in elastin and water content all lead to altered tendon stiffness. Diabetes accelerates the changes seen in aging tendons.[34] Physical activity has been shown to increase the cross-sectional area of tendons, while enhancing collagen turnover and remodeling.[10] Individuals who continue to exercise and incorporate flexibility and eccentric strength training slow the decline in flexibility otherwise seen with aging.[23]

Bone Changes

Bone mineral density (BMD) decreases, the cortex becomes thinner, adipose is deposited in marrow, and decreased osteoblast activity are all common age-related changes seen in bone. Women are affected earlier and more significantly than men.[7] In fact, women start losing BMD in their 30s and lose it a rate twice that of men.[35] Exercise is an important part of maintaining bone health.[36] Physical exercise, including resistance, aerobic, and endurance training, have all been shown help maintain and improve bone health.[35,37] Much focus has previously been placed on weight-bearing activity as promoting bone remodeling, but more recent research has shown that resistive exercises play an equivalent, or perhaps greater role, than weight-bearing activities in the management of osteoporosis.[38]

Cartilage Changes

Cartilage relies on joint loading and the fluid dynamics of synovial fluid for nutrition and removal of metabolic waste. Chondrocytes and extracellular matrix proteins experience little cell turnover so may be less resistant to aging than other tissues. In addition, increased oxidative stress and decreased growth factor found in aging cartilage may contribute to the development of osteoarthritis.[39] Decreased joint loading, such as that seen with even short-term immobilization, results in disuse atrophy and diminished metabolic activity of cartilage.[40]

Osteoarthritis (OA) is the most common source of musculoskeletal pain and disability in the older population.[21] Activities that subject the joints to high levels of impact and torsional loading can increase the risk of injury and cartilage degeneration.[41,42] Softening, fissuring, and fibrillation of the weight-bearing surfaces occur with repetitive joint loading and microtrauma to mechanically compromised articular cartilage. Individuals with early OA can benefit from regular exercise but should be advised to select activities that maintain joint motion and build strength with minimal joint loading.[41]

Skin and Other Tissue Changes

Thinning of the epidermal, dermal, and subcutaneous layers of the skin occurs with age.[7] This results in decreased resistance to sheer and friction, especially in the feet, which are subjected to impact forces and footwear. In addition, peripheral blood flow and autonomic nerve changes can contribute to dryness and decreased elasticity of the skin, further reducing its ability to resist tearing and ulceration, and to repair itself following insult.[43]

Other Physiologic Changes

There are other physiologic changes that can be less obvious in aging patients but also are important to consider for the sports medicine practitioner.

Inflammation generally increases with age, which results in prolonged inflammatory reactions in infections and delayed healing after injury. One group of researchers referred to this phenomenon as "inflamm-aging."[44] Inappropriate inflammatory responses to muscle injury could explain long-term deterioration of muscle mass and function in the elderly.[45] Although researchers are unsure of the causes of inflammation in older adults, they speculate that exercise and diet modifications may be important in managing this condition in the future.

The use of nonsteroidal anti-inflammatory drugs is more potentially problematic in older adults. The risk of gastrointestinal complications is higher and adverse events are more common with age.[46]

Issues related to hydration also can become more significant with age. Older individuals are more likely to become dehydrated and or suffer electrolyte imbalances because the thirst mechanism is less sensitive, renal function is decreased, and the sweat response is impaired.[47,48] Altered hydration can in turn contribute to decreased ability to thermoregulate and to regulate cardiopulmonary function and negatively affects performance.[49] Older adults should be made aware of these changes and encouraged to maintain fluid levels by drinking before they become thirsty, while not overhydrating.

OLDER ADULTS AND INJURY

Currently 12% of the US population is 65 and older and the aged population is expected to grow to 18% by 2030. Approximately 2 million patients older than 65 seek medical attention for athletic-based injury yearly.[50] Despite the increased emphasis on physical activity in older adults, there are few studies on injury rates and epidemiology.

The incidence of overuse injuries is higher and acute injuries are lower in older athletes than younger athletes.[25,26] Most acute injuries are related to falls or slips. Finnish researchers found that of the injuries sustained in athletes aged 70 to 81 during a 10-year period, 75% were to the lower extremity. The knee and foot/ankle were the most common sites at 20% and 19%, respectively.[51] Matheson and colleagues,[52] in a retrospective survey of 1407 injuries caused by physical activity, found that older individuals sustained more foot injuries whereas younger individuals were more likely to sustain knee injuries. Their study showed that injury cases decreased in the advancing age groups but they concluded that this was due to declining levels of sports participation and/or gravitation toward sports with lower injury risk with age. Fifty-two percent of the injured subjects in the survey reported their current diagnosis as an exacerbation of a previous problem.

This raises an interesting consideration: older adults, probably more so than younger adults, not only have to be cautious of new injuries but also of their previous injuries. This may require that they decrease the intensity of their athletic activities and/ or seek out other forms of exercise that allow them to remain active without increasing their risk for reinjury. For example, those who habitually run may need to decrease their running mileage or speed or transition to cycling and or swimming due to chronic knee injuries or OA.

The benefits of physical activity are broad and are linked to decreased functional decline with age and increased quality of life. Aging involves a number of physiologic changes that can be delayed or partially offset with exercise. Medical practitioners need to respect the significant physiologic and physical differences of their older patients. Although physical activity increases the risk of musculoskeletal injury, inactivity is a greater risk to the aging population's health. Sports medicine clinicians can and should educate and encourage their older patients to remain as active as possible to promote successful aging.

REFERENCES

1. National Council on Aging. Available at: NCOA.ORG. Accessed August 2, 2014.
2. Astrand PO. Exercise physiology of the mature athlete. In: Sutton J, Brock RM, editors. Sports medicine for the mature athlete. Indianapolis (IN): Benchmark Press; 1986. p. 3–13.

3. Jokl P, Sethi PM, Cooper AJ. Master's performance in the New York City marathon 1983–1999. Br J Sports Med 2004;38(4):408–12.
4. Kuland DN. The injured athlete. Philadelphia: J.B. Lippincott Co; 1982.
5. McCardle WD, Katch FJ, Katch VL. Exercise physiology—energy, nutrition and human performance. 2nd edition. Philadelphia: Lea & Febiger; 1986.
6. Siegel AJ, Warhol MJ, Lang G. Muscle injury and repair in ultra-long distance runners. In: Sutton J, Brock RM, editors. Sports medicine for the mature athlete. Indianapolis (IN): Benchmark Press; 1986. p. 35–43.
7. Menard D, Stanish WD. The aging athlete. Am J Sports Med 1989;17(2):187–96.
8. Hessert MJ, Gugliucci MR, Pierce HR. Functional fitness: maintaining or improving function for elders with chronic diseases. Fam Med 2005;37(7):472–6.
9. Montoye HJ, Van Huss WD, Olson H, et al. Study of the longevity and morbidity of college athletes. J Am Med Assoc 1956;162(12):1132–4.
10. National Institute on Aging Exercise Program. Available at: http://go4life.nia.nih.gov/. Accessed August 2, 2014.
11. Chen AL, Mears SC, Hawkins RJ. Orthopaedic care of the aging athlete. J Am Acad Orthop Surg 2005;13(6):407–16.
12. Cotman CW, Berchtold NC, Christie LA. Exercise builds brain health: key roles of growth factor cascades and inflammation. Trends Neurosci 2007;30(9):464–72.
13. Kramer AF, Erickson KI, Colcombe SJ. Exercise, cognition, and the aging brain. J Appl Physiol (1985) 2006;101(4):1237–42.
14. Weuve J, Kang JH, Manson JE, et al. Physical activity, including walking, and cognitive function in older women. J Am Med Assoc 2004;292:1454–61.
15. Heyn P, Abreu BC, Ottenbacher KJ, et al. The effects of exercise training on elderly persons with cognitive impairment and dementia: a meta-analysis. Arch Phys Med Rehabil 2004;85:1694–704.
16. Larson EB, Wang L, Bowen JD, et al. Exercise is associated with reduced risk for incident dementia among persons 65 years of age and older. Ann Intern Med 2006;144:73–81.
17. Rovio S, Helkala EL, Viitanen M, et al. Leisure time physical activity at midlife and the risk of dementia and Alzheimer's disease. Lancet Neurol 2005;4:705–11.
18. Sidney KH, Shephard RJ, Harrison JE. Endurance training and body composition of the elderly. Am J Clin Nutr 1977;30(3):326–33.
19. Hawkins SA, Wiswell RA, Marcell TJ. Exercise and the master athlete—a model of successful aging? J Gerontol A Biol Sci Med Sci 2003;58(11):1009–11.
20. Tanaka H, Seals DR. Endurance exercise performance in Masters athletes: age-associated changes and underlying physiological mechanisms. J Physiol 2008;586:55–63.
21. Morley JE. The aging athlete [editorial]. J Gerontol A Biol Sci Med Sci 2000;55(11):627–9.
22. Herring SA, Kibler WB, Putukian M, et al. Selected issues for the master athlete and the team physician: a consensus statement. Med Sci Sports Exerc 2010;42(4):820–33.
23. Dorfman LJ, Bosley TM. Age-related changes in peripheral and central nerve conduction in man. Neurology 1979;29:38–44.
24. Covey A, Jokl P. Qualitative performance of the aging athlete. J Med Sci Tennis 2009;14(3):5–15.
25. Tennstedt S, Howland J, Lachman M, et al. A randomized, controlled trial of a group intervention to reduce fear of falling and associated activity restriction in older adults. J Gerontol B Psychol Sci Soc Sci 1998;53(6):P384–92.
26. DeHaven KE, Lintner DM. Athletic injuries: comparison by age, sport, and gender. Am J Sports Med 1986;14:218–24.

27. Kannus P, Niittymaki S, Jarvinen M, et al. Sports injuries in elderly athletes: a three year prospective, controlled study. Age Ageing 1989;4:263–70.
28. Wolfson L, Whipple R, Derby C, et al. Balance and strength training in older adults: intervention gains and Tai Chi maintenance. J Am Geriatr Soc 1996;44(5):498–506.
29. Nevitt MC, Cummings SR, Kidd S, et al. Risk factors for recurrent non-syncopal falls: a prospective study. JAMA 1989;261:2663–8.
30. Murry PM, Duthie EH, Gambert SR. Age-related changes in knee muscle strength in normal women. J Gerontol 1985;40:275–80.
31. Stalberg E, Borges O, Ericson M. The quadriceps muscle in 20 to 70-year old subjects: relationships between knee extension torque, electrophysiologic parameters and muscle fiber characteristics. Muscle Nerve 1989;12:382–9.
32. Evans WJ, Hurley BF. Age, gender, and muscular strength. J Gerontol A Biol Sci Med Sci 1995;50(Special Issue):41–4.
33. Maffulli N, Barrass V, Ewen S. Light microscopic histology of Achilles tendon ruptures. Am J Sports Med 2000;28(6):857–63.
34. Hamlin CR, Kohn RR, Luschin JH. Apparent accelerated aging of human collagen in diabetes mellitus. Diabetes 1975;24(10):902–4.
35. Kaplan FS, Hayes WC, Keaveny TM, et al. Form and function of bone. In: Simon SR, editor. Orthopaedic basic science. Rosemont (IL): American Academy of Orthopaedic Surgeons; 1994. p. 127–84.
36. Kai MC, Anderson M, Lau E. Exercise interventions: defusing the world's osteoporosis time bomb. Bull World Health Organ 2003;81(11):827–30.
37. Layne JE, Nelson ME. The effects of progressive resistance training on bone density: a review. Med Sci Sports Exerc 1999;31(1):25–30.
38. Swezey RL. Exercise for osteoporosis—is walking enough? The case for site specificity and resistive exercise. Spine (Phila Pa 1976) 1996;21(23):2809–13.
39. Loeser RF Jr. Aging cartilage and osteoarthritis—what's the link? Sci Aging Knowledge Environ 2004;2004(29):pe31.
40. Hall MC. Cartilage changes after experimental relief of contact in the knee joint of the mature rat. Clin Orthop Relat Res 1969;64:64–76.
41. Vingard E, Alfredsson L, Goldie I, et al. Sports and osteoarthrosis of the hip: an epidemiologic study. Am J Sports Med 1993;21(2):195–200.
42. Buckwalter JA, Lane NE. Aging, sports, and osteoarthritis. Sports Med Arthrosc Rev 1996;4(3):276–87.
43. Farage MA, Miller KW, Berardesca E, et al. Clinical implications of aging skin. Am J Clin Dermatol 2009;10(2):73–86.
44. Franceschi C, Capri M, Monti D, et al. Inflammaging and anti-inflammaging: a systemic perspective on aging and longevity emerged from studies in humans. Mech Ageing Dev 2007;128:92–105.
45. Peake J, Della Gatta P, Cameron-Smith D. Aging and its effects on inflammation in skeletal muscle at rest and following exercise-induced muscle injury. Am J Physiol Regul Integr Comp Physiol 2010;298(6):R1485–95.
46. Barkin RL, Beckerman M, Blum SL, et al. Should nonsteroidal anti-inflammatory drugs (NSAIDs) be prescribed to the older adult? Drugs Aging 2010;27(10):775–89.
47. Kenney WL, Chiu P. Influence of age on thirst and fluid intake. Med Sci Sports Exerc 2001;33(9):1524–32.
48. Phillips PA, Rolls BJ, Ledingham JG, et al. Reduced thirst after water deprivation in healthy elderly men. N Engl J Med 1984;311(12):753–9.
49. Rolls BJ, Phillips PA. Aging and disturbances of thirst and fluid balance. Nutr Rev 1990;48(3):137–44.

50. Heinkinj K. The geriatric athlete. Chapter 42. In: Karageanes SJ, editor. Principles of manual sports medicine. Philadelphia: Lippincott Williams and Wilkins; 2005. p. 628–40.

51. Kallinen M, Alen M. Sports-related injuries in elderly men still active in sports. Br J Sports Med 1994;28(1):52–5.

52. Matheson GO, MacIntyre JG, Taunton JE, et al. Musculoskeletal injuries associated with physical activity in older adults. Med Sci Sports Exerc 1989;21(4): 379–85.

Principles of Rehabilitation and Return to Sports Following Injury

Magali Fournier, DPM

KEYWORDS

- Athletic injuries • Return to sport • Rehabilitation • Sports medicine

KEY POINTS

- Rehabilitation of athlete after lower extremity injury requires thorough evaluation and understanding of the demands of the sport.
- Few protocols exist to guide the physician in helping the athlete returning to sport.
- Protocols and plan of care must be individualized and constantly reevaluated to maximize return to sport and decrease the incidence of re-injury.
- A multidisciplinary team is often required to better treat athletes and permit a prompt return to sport.

INTRODUCTION

Injuries to the foot and ankle during athletic activities are a common occurrence, representing approximately 25% of all sports injuries seen in sports medicine specialty clinics.[1] Elite and recreational athletes who suffer from such injury will be faced with the inability to participate in sports, and for professional athletes, such injury can lead to a lack of income. Whether conservative measure or surgical correction is necessary for the treatment of the athlete, a well-planned rehabilitation program is essential to ensure a successful treatment and return to sport. The most efficient and successful treatment plan can be futile if the athlete is not properly reintroduced to his or her sport.

Treating athletes successfully should surpass usual treatment protocol. An added step needs to be implemented because the physical demands on an athlete's lower extremity is beyond the tasks of daily living; it requires the ability to endure strenuous physical loads that are specialized for each individual's sports. It is therefore imperative to have a thorough understanding of the necessary steps to take to get a patient and athlete beyond healing, and return the athlete to his or her sport.

Disclosure: Nothing to disclose, no conflict of interest reported.
Departments of Orthopaedics, Podiatry and Sports Medicine, Gundersen Health Systems, 1900 south avenue, LaCrosse, WI 54601, USA
E-mail address: mfournie@gundersenhealth.org

Clin Podiatr Med Surg 32 (2015) 261–268
http://dx.doi.org/10.1016/j.cpm.2014.11.009
0891-8422/15/$ – see front matter © 2015 Elsevier Inc. All rights reserved.

podiatric.theclinics.com

Instituting a rehabilitation program for an athlete recovering from an injury is imperative, but unfortunately, specific protocols are difficult to find in the published literature. There is a significant lack of clinical evidence and studies analyzing proper protocols for the return of an athlete safely to his or her sport within a timely manner. This can cause frustration for the patient, the athletic trainers, coaches, and physician. The heterogeneity of sports injuries, the number of sports, and the number of lower extremity sports-related injuries make it difficult to carry out meaningful clinical trials. There are several suggested protocols, but few are validated, which can make it difficult for a sports physician to ensure safe return to sport for his/her patient.

In order to have a better understanding of the steps to take, it is important to, first and foremost, understand the basic science behind healing tissues. The phases of rehabilitation closely match the phases of healing, which determine the athlete's stage of healing and whether or not he or she is ready to advance to the next phase. It is also important to realize that each individual has his or her own healing rate. The healing rate is determined by several factors, including the athlete's degree of injury, prior level of conditioning, age, type of sport, time between the initial symptoms and time of treatment, but also motivation level, access to specific treatment facility, and social system, such as coaches and athletic trainers. The treating physician needs to be flexible and must do close follow-up with the injured athlete to ascertain if efficient progress is being made in the right direction.

This article presents an overview of the current existing data about protocols aimed to help the physician in the proper return of their patients safely and in a timely manner to their sports after an injury and/or surgery has occurred.

GOALS OF REHABILITATION

Rehabilitation after a sport injury is the process needed for a timely, safe return to sport participation, whether the patient is a recreational or professional athlete. Restoration of the preinjury function serves as the primary goal, or baseline objective, but it is to be understood that some patients may never achieve preinjury level of sports participation. Therefore, every rehabilitation protocol or program should be individualized to the specific patient's need.[2] Even though the protocol should be individualized, it should also follow general principles outlined. They all share basic goals, which are as follow[3]

1. Decrease pain
2. Reduction or elimination of edema
3. Restoration of unrestricted range of motion
4. Regain strength necessary for the specific sport
5. Improve gait pattern and close kinetic chain motion
6. Minimize risk of reinjury
7. Sports-specific agility drills
8. Maintain cardiovascular fitness

Rehabilitation becomes a process of applying stress to healing tissues until the body can sustain a stress similar to the demand of the sport. Therefore, a thorough understanding of the biology and the physiology of the healing tissues is imperative in order to comprehend and safely implement the phases of rehabilitation. One cannot advance to a higher, more aggressive level if the stressed tissue is not mature or healed enough. The phases of rehabilitation are closely related to the phases of tissue healing:

1. Acute phase/inflammatory stage
2. Reparative phase/intermediate stage
3. Return to sport/remodeling stage

A rehabilitation program, whether from a conservative or surgical management, should follow the previously described phases.[1] The physician's role is to direct such a program based on the physical examination findings and determine when the rehabilitation should be advanced to the next level or even slowed to let some of the scar tissue heal. These determinations are based on comparative findings of the physical examination.

With every patient presenting with a sport injury, a specific goal-oriented, step-wise approach should be instituted. After a thorough history & physical (H&P), the following steps should take place

1. Have a precise diagnosis (imperative in order to have a precise treatment plan). Additional imaging studies or tests should be performed if needed.
2. Know the demand of the sport; is there any athletic gear to take into consideration? One must also know and understand biomechanical requirements of the specific sport.
3. Form a plan with time frame and expectations. Communicate; it is imperative to discuss with the patient so that she or he understands realistic expectations. In turn, it will help him or her make plans with regards to determining future participation schedule, loss of season, loss of income, or other considerations.
4. Form/have a team. It often involves many professionals, each with specific roles to help the athlete through his or her recovery. It is necessary to have proper communication so that everybody understands the constraints, severity, and anticipated time frame. It may include: athletic trainers, physical therapist, nutritionists, coaches, and psychologists.
5. Be familiar with any specific governing rules and regulations to consider regarding participation that may affect the return to sport.

BASIC SCIENCES

As previously mentioned, the phases of rehabilitation closely follow the stages of healing tissue and should be understood in order to have a better understanding of the process that each athlete must go through before advancing to the next level.

Healing stages include

1. Inflammatory stage
2. Reparative stage
3. Remodeling stage

Inflammatory Stage: Hematoma Formation

The healing process starts with a hematoma formation at the site of injury. This stage is characterized by cellular and vascular responses to an injury, which in turn, release inflammatory mediators creating vasodilation, leading to edema, ecchymosis, pain, and reduced function. Hematoma formation at the site of the injury will later provide the matrix for scar tissue formation.

Reparative Stage: Collagen Synthesis

This stage involves the necrosis of the damaged tissue and synthesis of collagen through fibroblast proliferation. The hematoma is being replaced by a fibrous matrix. Collagen synthesis begins within the first week and will reach its maximum level after about 4 weeks. At this stage, the formed product is a poorly organized matrix not strong enough or suitable to sustain the stress of the sport.

Remodeling: Collagen Organization

This stage results in reorganizing the new collagen fibrils in order to gain mechanical strength. It is the stage that reshapes and strengthens tissue. Collagen maturation and remodeling begin in the second to third week, and by 28 days, most of the fibrils are organized, leading to an increase in strength. The collagen will continue to mature and can do so up until 1 year after the injury. Therefore, this stage may extend for years in some patients.

PHASES OF REHABILITATION

Phases coincide with general principles and time frames of healing tissue. It is also important to understand there is no absolute transition from 1 phase to another, and phases may overlap. It is therefore imperative to have proper intervals between clinical follow-ups to assess the correct progression of the recovering athlete.[4] Each phase has specific goals to achieve before advancing to the next, rather than being based on a specific time frame. A clinician must be willing to adapt depending of the individual's progression and healing time. There are 3 basic phases:

1. Acute phase/inflammatory stage
2. Reparative phase/intermediate stage
3. Return to sport/remodeling stage

Acute Phase

Goals in this phase include

- Preventing excess edema
- Preventing excess hematoma formation
- Increasing tensile strength
- Controlling pain

This phase starts from the moment the injury occurs to the moment the edema is controlled. Initial treatment of the acute injury follows the RICE (rest, ice, compression, elevation) principle in order to reduce pain, bleeding, and edema, which in turn, reduces permanent scar tissue.[5] The primary objective and function of ice is to reduce inflammation and pain, by causing vasoconstriction and slowing the down the nerve conduction velocity.[6,7] Cryotherapy is most effective within the first 72 hours after the injury but can be continued as long as several months thereafter. Icing should be closely monitored, because it has the potential for thermal injury. Elevation and compression will reduce hydrostatic pressure thus decrease the edema. At this stage, early range of motion can be initiated but often presents a dilemma, as it is the topic of debates and controversies. Studies show that early immobilization helps avoid further tissue damage and helps reduce scar tissue formation, but concurrently, allows the scar tissue to regain strength to sustain future applied forces. This in turns prevents reinjury and is an important step to consider. Obviously, the amount of tension applied must not overcome ultimate load of failure and must be closely monitored. However, if immobilization is carried out for an extended period of time, this can lead to excess fibrosis and adhesions, atrophy of the muscle and loss of strength. The period of immobilization should be carried for up to 3 to 7 days after which, gentle range of motion can be performed.[4,5] One should be aware of the adverse effects of immobilization, if carried out beyond the acute phase; these effects can include: muscle atrophy (between 0.5% and 1% per day for the quadriceps muscle) and structural changes in connective tissue leading to decreased range of motion and deconditioning.[8] A recent systematic review and meta-analysis by Huang showed that early weight bearing, within 1 to 2 weeks after surgical treatment of acute Achilles tendon ruptures, led to better functional outcome and more rapid recovery without increasing the complication rate.[9] A similar systematic review on return to sport after ankle fractures also demonstrated that early weight bearing (at 1 week after injury) also leads to better functional outcome.[10] Therefore, a balance between early range of motion and immobilization must be achieved.

Reparative Phase

The goals of this phase are to

- Regain strength
- Regain range of motion
- Prepare the athlete for the physical demands of the return to sport phase
- Continue to maintain conditioning of the noninjured area (cross-training)

This phase starts once the edema is controlled. At this time, connective tissue is still immature but can sustain a certain amount of stress, which is necessary in order to regain strength. As described by Wolf's law, injured bone and tissue stressed in a controlled manner will lead to further healing and hypertrophy, which in turn will lead to strength. The focus of this phase is to regain flexibility and strength of the injured site, all while maintaining some type of cardiovascular fitness. This phase ends once range of motion of the injured limb is pain-free, and most of the range of motion has been regained.

Return to Sport Phase

The goals of this phase are

- Sports-specific demands
- Sports-specific skills
- Adequate range of motion
- Symmetry
- Agility drills
- General conditioning
- Bench mark test

This phase starts when the patient has regained full range of motion and muscle strength, as well as appropriate proprioception. It is often a frustrating time period, as the patient is mostly symptom-free, but a gradual and controlled return to sport is vital to prevent reoccurrence of the injury. It is imperative at this stage to progress the athlete through a series of functional testing and drills specific to his or her sport, to ensure a controlled, gradual and safe return to sport. It is often easy for the athlete to want to get back at his or her preinjury level and being impatient. External support such as braces, taping, or orthotics may be used to help the patient regain pain-free activity, and these supports can be used for as long as needed. When the athlete is symptom-free, the latter portion of this phase should incorporate agility drills, plyometric exercises, and sports-specific skills.[11]

WHEN IS THE ATHLETE READY?

Rehabilitating the athlete back to sport in a timely manner is the goal of any successful injury management. One should want to minimize the time needed, yet, too early of a return to sport can also mean a risk for reinjury. Having the knowledge of a proposed and sound return to sport protocol and knowing how to execute it can be 2 different and separate matters.[12] A study published by Gajhede-Knutson in 2013 showed an increase in reoccurrence rate of Achilles tendon disorders in elite male European football players after a period of recovery less than 10 days.[13] As previously mentioned, studies are lacking that clearly define time frame and specific criteria for the foot and ankle injuries. Several studies are available regarding objective criteria after knee surgeries, specifically after anterior cruciate ligament reconstructions. Saxena and colleagues published guidelines and studies discussing effective return to sport time frames and protocols. One study in particular outlined a protocol and specific criteria for a safe return to sport after having an operated Achilles tendon. His findings showed that it is safe for the patient to return to activities once he or she demonstrates the ability to perform[14-16]:

1. 5 sets of 25 single-legged concentric heel raises
2. Symmetry of calf girth within 5 mm of the contralateral side
3. Ankle range of motion with 5° of the contralateral side

A systematic review was also published presenting objective criteria used to allow release to return to sport, for patient who underwent anterior cruciate ligament reconstruction. One can extrapolate these findings to the lower extremity and used them as guidelines. The review outlined the following criteria, based on the review of 21 studies over a 10 year span and determined that muscle strength, limb symmetry, and range of motion were criteria being used for safe return to sport and showing a low rate of reinjury.[17]

Several functional tests have been described and are routinely used during physical therapy that aim, not only to determine when the patient is ready, but also to prepare the patient to the specific demands of his or her sport. Again, most of those tests have been validated in the knee rehabilitation literature, but these tests evaluate the entire lower extremity kinetic chain and again, can be easily extrapolated to the foot and ankle.[18,19] Functional tests are also used as baseline and to monitor adequate progression. The quality of the motion is also important, in addition to how many can be performed.

Here are some examples of functional performance tests:

- Single-leg hop
- Vertical jump
- Hop for distance
- Stair hop

The uninjured leg should be tested first, followed by the injured side, performed after a period of warm up. The American College of Sports Medicine is a well-known resource, and it publishes a consensus statement aimed at guiding physicians with decision making when returning an athlete to sport. The statement was developed by the collaborative efforts of several professional associations and is revised every few years.[20] The latest consensus statement was published in 2012. It serves as a guide to help guide physicians with medically clearing an athlete back to sport. It outlines goals of returning to sport, processes, and protocols. It is an easily accessible guide that one can refer to when questions or concerns arise.

PSYCHOLOGICAL ASPECT OF THE ATHLETIC INJURY

Numerous studies have examined the psychological factors associated with sports-related injuries. Sports psychology as a recognized specialty began in 1960.[8,21,22]

When an athlete is injured, there is an immediate assessment of the actual physical injury and the impact it will have on the athlete's participation in sport. One also needs to realize that sport itself is often a primary coping mechanism of an athlete's stressful life events. Not only is the injury causing anxiety, but the loss of sport as an outlet and coping mechanism will in turn, create even further stress. Athletic injuries can lead to

- Loss of coping mechanism through sport
- Loss of social interaction surrounding sport
- Loss of self-value and recognition from others

Physicians need to be aware and mindful of their patient's mental well-being and be ready to engage additional resources to help. In addition to helping the athlete with grieving, the field of sport psychology can help directly in rehabilitation. Certain techniques can be used such as visualization (imaging), goal setting, and mental rehearsal of the actual physical athletic activity. The athlete may also need help in getting rid of negative thoughts or irrational fears brought by the actual trauma of the injury, a process termed cognitive restructuring.[21] It is therefore important for the athlete to have a social system composed of family, friends, teammates, athletic trainers, coaches, and the sports psychologist to help directly with his or her return to sport, in addition to the medical and physical aspects.

The treating physician may also play a part in the psychological aspect of a sport injury. The physician may help by educating the athlete about his or her injury and condition, which in turn, allows the athlete to foster a sense of control and understanding. Giving the athlete goals to work toward and benchmarks may also provide motivation. The athlete can feel as if he or she is actively participating, engaging directly in his or her recovery. Creating a healthy and trusting rapport with the athlete provides a healthy environment for both the treating physician and the athlete and is an important aspect to recognize for the successful management of injuries.

SUMMARY

Returning to sport after treating an athletic injury can be challenging with the goal to returning the athlete to his or her preinjury level in the shortest amount of time without further risk of injury. Treatment guidelines and protocols for the lower extremity athletic injury rehabilitation are sparse. This article has outlined the phases the athlete requires to successfully achieve a safe return to sport, based on the current available information.

REFERENCES

1. Hawson ST. Physical therapy and rehabilitation of the foot and ankle in the athlete. Clin Podiatr Med Surg 2011;28:189–201.
2. Konin J. Introduction to rehabilitation. Clin Sports Med 2010;29:1–4.
3. Hudson Z. Rehabilitation and return to play after foot and ankle injuries in athletes. Sports Med Arthrosc Rev 2009;17(3):203–7.
4. Mendiguchia J, Brughelli M. A return-to-sport algorithm for acute hamstring injuries. Phys Ther Sport 2011;12:2–14.
5. Järvinen TA, Järvinen TL, Kääinen M, et al. Muscle injuries: optimizing recovery. Best Pract Res Clin Rheumatol 2007;21(2):317–31.
6. Porter DA, Schon LC. Baxter's the foot and ankle in sport textbook. 2nd edition. Philadelphia: Mosby Elsevier; 2008.
7. Delee JC, Drez D, Miller MD. Delee & Drez's orthopedic sports medicine textbook. 3rd edition. Philadelphia: Saunders Elsevier; 2009.

8. Andrews JR, Harrelson GL, Wilk KE. Physical rehabilitation of the injured Athlete textbook. 4th edition. Philadelphia: Saunders Elsevier; 2012.
9. Huang J, Wang C, Ma X, et al. Rehabilitation regimen after surgical treatment of acute tendon ruptures: a systematic review with meta-analysis. Am J Sports Med 2014. [Epub ahead of print].
10. Del Buono A, Smith R, Coco M, et al. Return to sports after ankle fractures: a systematic review. Br Med Bull 2013;106:179–91.
11. Hudson Z. Rehabilitation and return to play after foot and ankle injuries in athletes. Sports Med Arthrosc 2009;17(3):203–7.
12. Chinn L, Hertel J. Rehabilitation of ankle and foot injuries in athletes. Clin Sports Med 2010;29:157–67.
13. Gajhede-Knudsen M, Ekstrand J, Magnusson H, et al. Recurrence of Achilles tendon injury in elite male football players is more common after early return to play: an 11-year follow-up of the UEFA champions league injury study. Br J Sports Med 2013;47:763–8.
14. Saxena A. Return to athletic activity after foot and ankle surgery: a preliminary report on select procedures. J Foot Ankle Surg 2000;39(2):114–9.
15. Saxena A, Ewen B, Maffulli N. Rehabilitation of the operated Achilles tendon: parameters for predicting return to activity. J Foot Ankle Surg 2011;50:37–40.
16. Saxena A, Cheung S. Pushing the envelope: case studies on how fast you can and cannot return the elite athlete to running. Clin Podiatr Med Surg 2001; 18(2):319–28.
17. Barber-Westin SD, Noyes FR. Objective criteria for return to athletics after anterior cruciate ligament reconstruction and subsequent reinjury rates: a systematic review. The Physician and Sports Medicine 2011;39(3):100–10.
18. Cook JL, Purdam CR. Rehabilitation of the lower limb tendinopathies. Clin Sports Med 2003;22:777–89.
19. Herrington L, Myer G, Horsley I. Task based rehabilitation protocol for elite athletes following anterior cruciate ligament reconstruction: a clinical commentary. Phys Ther Sport 2013;14:188–98.
20. Herring SA, Kibler WB, Putukian M. The team physician and the return-to-play decision: a consensus statement- 2012 update. Med Sci Sports Exerc 2012;44(12): 2446–8.
21. Ahern DK, Lohr BA. Psychosocial factors in sports injury rehabilitation. Clin Sports Med 1997;16(4):755–68.
22. Williams RA, Appaneal RN. Social support and sport injury. Athletic Therapy Today 2010;15:46–9.

Index

Note: Page numbers of article titles are in **boldface** type.

A

Achilles tendinopathy, and plantar fasciopathy, emerging technologies for, **183–193**
   extracorporeal shock wave therapy in, 183–187
Achilles tendon, rupture of, 222–224
Adults, older, age-related physical and physiologic changes in, 254–257
     and injury, 257
     as prone to overuse injuries, 254
     bone changes in, 256
     cartilage changes in, 256
     muscle changes in, 255
     neurologic changes in, 255
     physically active, and aging athletes, considerations for treating, **253–260**
       exercise and, 253–254
     physiologic changes in, 256–257
     skin and tissue changes in, 256
     tendon changes in, 255–256
     vascular changes in, 255
     weight gain and, 254
American Academy of Podiatric Sports Medicine, birth of, sports medicine and, 174
American College of Sports Medicine, podiatrists and, 179
Ankle, lateral, ligaments of, clinical tests for assessment of, 219–220, 221
     sprain of ligaments involved in, 220
   musculoskeletal examination of, 219–226
Ankle instability, chronic, 196
Ankle sprain, ankle braces in, 210–211
   as common injury, 195
   bracing and orthoses in, 210–211
   evaluation and treatment in, 196–197
   foot orthoses in, 210
   functional performance testing following, 201–205
   heel rocker rest for, 208
   lateral hop test and forward hop test following, 205–207
   manual tests for stability following, 208–209
   recovery following, self-reported variables on, 199–202
   recovery from, protection of ankle during, 197–198
   rehabilitation following, 197
   restoration of neuromuscular control following, 198
   restoration of sports-specific skills following, 210
   return to play after, **195–215**
   single leg stance for time following, 207–208
   strength deficits following, 198–199

Clin Podiatr Med Surg 32 (2015) 269–273
http://dx.doi.org/10.1016/S0891-8422(15)00012-9
0891-8422/15/$ – see front matter © 2015 Elsevier Inc. All rights reserved.

Moving?

Make sure your subscription moves with you!

To notify us of your new address, find your **Clinics Account Number** (located on your mailing label above your name), and contact customer service at:

Email: journalscustomerservice-usa@elsevier.com

800-654-2452 (subscribers in the U.S. & Canada)
314-447-8871 (subscribers outside of the U.S. & Canada)

Fax number: 314-447-8029

Elsevier Health Sciences Division
Subscription Customer Service
3251 Riverport Lane
Maryland Heights, MO 63043

*To ensure uninterrupted delivery of your subscription, please notify us at least 4 weeks in advance of move.

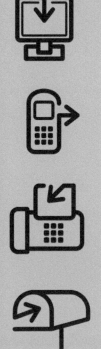

Printed and bound by CPI Group (UK) Ltd, Croydon, CR0 4YY

03/10/2024

01040494-0015